PLANT-BASED HIGH-PROTEIN COOKBOOK

How to Lose Weight, Build Muscle, and Transform Your Body

Charles Baker

TABLE OF CONTENTS

Chapter 11: It's Dinner Time! Whole Food Meals to Aid Recovery

Chapter 12: Let's Get Saucy - Flavor Boosters and Sauces for Exciting Meals

INTRODUCTION

Greetings! I would like to congratulate you for taking action to improve your health and increase your lifespan. Please allow me to take this time to tell you why you are absolutely doing the right thing by considering a plant-based diet.

In 2015, the World Health Organization labeled processed red meat a carcinogen, which increases the risk of rectum or colon cancer by 18 percent. However, processed red meat is not the only battle you are fighting. The consumption of both white and red meat can cause significant health challenges.

A 2014 study conducted by Harvard University discovered that just one serving of red meat per day during adolescence increased the risk of pre-menopausal breast cancer by 22 percent. The same level of red meat consumption in adulthood increased the risk of breast cancer by 18 percent (Farvid MS, 2014).

Meat, eggs, and dairy products all contain saturated fats and cholesterol, which contribute to the top killers in the world: Heart attack, cancer, stroke, and diabetes. Saturated fat is present in all meats, including chicken, turkey, and fish, even when cooked without the skin.

The American Diabetes Association reported that large consumptions of animal protein increased the risk of developing diabetes by 22 percent (ADA, 2014). Breast cancer and conditions related to cognitive declines, such as dementia and Alzheimer's disease, are said to be linked to saturated fat.

The good news is that there is a healthy alternative to eating meat and processed foods, and that is a plant-based diet.

In 2015, I was diagnosed with type II diabetes. I was severely overweight, addicted to sugar, and depressed. My diagnosis was a blessing in disguise because it has transformed my life for the better. I refused to accept that taking insulin permanently was the only solution. As I began to research the disease and communicate with other people who had healed themselves from the condition, I learned that diabetes was diet-related, and plant-based nutrition was one of the most effective cures. I am not a doctor, and I wouldn't advise you to take my word for it without going out and doing your own research; however, here are some of the studies that convinced me I was on the right path:

> A study published in JAMA Internal Medicine found that one of the main factors in controlling blood sugar levels is a plant-based diet (Frank B. Hu et al., 2019)

> A study published in the Journal of Geriatric Cardiology reported that a plant-based diet was an effective tool for the treatment and management of type II diabetes (JCG, 2017)

> The BMJ Journal reported that a plant-based diet is the most effective nutrition plan for type II diabetes (Toumpanakis et al., 2018)

I started to notice a difference in my health within the first 30 days of being on a plant-based diet. Within two years, I was fully healed of type II diabetes. I also experienced several other improvements to my overall well-being:

- High energy levels
- Improved focus
- Better skin
- Thicker and shinier hair
- Weight loss

You might not have type II diabetes, but as you have read, there are many other benefits associated with a plant-based diet. In this book, you will gain in-depth knowledge about proper plant-based nutrition as well as a large selection of simple and delicious recipes.

There is no time like the present, if your health is failing due to dangerous processed foods, or you want to avoid becoming a victim of diet-related diseases, use this book to begin your journey to a healthier lifestyle today!

CHAPTER 1:
THE PRINCIPLE OF ENERGY BALANCE - FUNDAMENTAL KEYS TO SUCCESS

If you've been trying to shed those extra pounds, I am assuming you are familiar with the phrase "calories in, calories out." Calories are energy, and when you consume more than you burn, the body stores the excess as fat. Being overweight increases the risk of cancer, heart disease, and diabetes. Therefore, maintaining energy balance is essential.

What is Energy Balance?

Food calories consumed through food and drink are converted into energy and used to perform daily activities such as walking, running, cleaning, cooking, etc. "Energy in" refers to the food we eat, and "energy out" refers to calories used by the body. The relationship between the energy we take in, and the energy we put out indicates "energy balance," and it determines whether we lose or gain weight, or whether our weight remains the same. Energy balance must be maintained, and physical activity is a crucial part of the equation. The more physically active a person is, the more calories are burned. Weight remains the same when the calories consumed and burned are the same. When more calories are consumed than burned, it leads to weight gain.

Energy balance must be maintained daily. The best way to achieve this is through a consistently healthy diet and exercise. If you want to maintain a desirable weight, yoyo dieting is not the answer, but energy balance is.

Energy Balance in Real Life

The first step is to pay attention to your calorie intake; everything you eat has a nutrition label on the back, which makes it easy to count calories. According to the World Health Organization, the average adult should consume 2000 calories per day. Consuming the recommended daily intake of calories is not always easy to achieve; there are going to be some days when you consume more, and others when you consume less. The good news is that it's possible to balance out your energy intake and output.

Let's say a colleague is leaving work and the office is going out for a meal and a drink. You can lower your calorie intake a few days before to make up for the additional calories you are going to consume. Or you can intensify your workouts before and after the party to burn the extra calories.

If you've got kids, the same applies. If they have a birthday party to go to or any other activity which involves consuming more calories, increase their physical activity, or give them fewer calories before the event.

CHAPTER 2:
CARBS AND FATS - WHAT THEY ARE AND HOW THEY IMPACT PERFORMANCE

For athletes to achieve energy balance, they also require the right number of proteins, carbohydrates, and fats. Macronutrients provide fuel for energy expenditure and athletes need to consume them in adequate quantities. If not, it limits the availability of energy.

Athletic Performance and Carbohydrates

Carbohydrates are an essential nutrient in an athlete's diet; they enable the body to perform to its optimal standard during physical activity for two reasons:

1. Energy: The brain and body require energy to function; when carbohydrates are consumed and digested, they are broken down into glucose, which is stored in the muscles and liver and used as fuel during physical activity. According to Michael Gleeson, Ph.D., and Jeukendrup, Ph.D., several studies indicate that fueling the body with carbohydrates for

45 minutes or more can improve athletic performance and endurance.

2. <u>Muscle Gain</u>: When there is a limited supply of glucose in the body, other nutrients such as muscle protein and fat are used as energy. When the muscles get the right amount of carbohydrates, protein can effectively perform its primary job of repairing and rebuilding muscle tissue, which boosts muscle gain.

Carbohydrates assist athletes in performing at their best by replenishing muscle glycogen stores, which is not possible on a low-carbohydrate, high-protein diet.

Fats: The Difference Between Good and Bad

During an athletic performance, the body's main source of energy comes from carbohydrates; however, when low-intensity workouts and extensive periods of athletic activity are performed, the main energy source is from fats.

Fat is an essential part of our diet; however, to enjoy the health benefits of fat, you must understand the difference between good and bad fats. Fats from meat and dairy products are called saturated fats, and they increase the amount of bad cholesterol (low-density lipoprotein, LDL) in the blood. Those who consume excessive amounts of saturated fats increase their risk of heart disease or stroke, states the American Heart Association. A vegan diet contains limited amounts of saturated fats; they are found in foods such as cocoa butter, palm oil, and coconuts. Therefore, it is advised that those on a plant-based diet refrain from eating plant-based foods high in saturated fats. If you are going to consume these foods, ensure that they make up under 30 percent of the fat you eat.

Many plant-based foods contain monounsaturated fats, which assist in lowering LDL cholesterol, which reduces the risk of stroke and heart disease. Foods containing monounsaturated fats include walnuts, Brazil nuts, and almonds, olive oil, avocados, and tahini.

Despite the negative effects of saturated fats, their main benefit is that they increase serotonin levels. Serotonin is an important hormone that plays a role in mood regulation and is known to alleviate depression, improve sleep, and reduce feelings of anxiety.

Finally, good fats enhance the bodies nutrient absorbing capabilities, with the main nutrients being vitamins A, D, and E; as fat-soluble vitamins, they are not absorbed by the body without the assistance of healthy fats. Vitamins A, D, and E are responsible for maintaining healthy skin, creating hormones, and boosting the immune system.

How to Consume Healthy Fats on a Vegan Diet

There are many ways you can consume healthy fats on a vegan diet; here are some of them:

1. Cook mushrooms, winter squash, and carrots in olive oil.
2. Eat nuts high in unsaturated fats such as almonds after a workout. Unsaturated fats are capable of reducing inflammation; therefore, you are likely to experience reduced muscle soreness.
3. Use flaxseeds instead of flaxseed oil, they are both rich in healthy fats, but flaxseeds are also high in fiber.
4. Increase your polyunsaturated fat intake to reduce high cholesterol levels.
5. Educate yourself about the foods that are rich in healthy fats.

CHAPTER 3:
THE POTENTIAL OF PROTEINS - WHY THEY'RE CRUCIAL FOR ATHLETES

The right nutrition is essential for athletes to perform at their best. They use excessive amounts of energy during long, intensive workouts; the body also experiences changes such as muscle damage. For the body to recover, it requires sufficient rest and nutrition, which enables the following:

- Muscle restoration and growth
- Limits the chance of illness and injury
- Gets the body ready for another intense workout

For the body to recover, it needs to replace lost sweat with electrolytes and fluids, protein to rebuild and repair muscle tissue, and carbohydrates to replenish glycogen. When it comes to recovery, protein is vital because athletes require a lot more than the average healthy person who does a limited amount of exercise.

Protein – How Much?

Athletes should consume protein 30-60 minutes after a workout to get the maximum glycogen stores and to enhance muscle protein synthesis. Between 30-60 minutes after a workout is a perfect time to restore energy with protein and carbs because protein accelerates the process of muscles converting carbohydrates into stored energy. However, if you are unable to refuel during this timeframe, just make sure you get some protein in with your snacks and meals throughout the day. Here are the recommended amounts of protein you should consume:

- 1 gram per pound: This amount of protein provides you with enough to build muscle.
- 0.82 grams per pound: There is a lot of speculation about whether 0.82 grams is enough protein to facilitate muscle growth; however, research suggests that it is, but it's the lowest amount you should consume.
- 1.5 grams: If you consistently go overboard with your cheat meals, 1.5 grams per pound of protein will be of benefit to you.

The extra protein will probably not result in increased gains; however, increasing your protein intake will do the following:

- Will keep you full for longer
- Eating more protein will force you to eat less junk because your food choices are restricted
- The thermic effect of food (TEF) suggests protein is not 4 kcal per gram but closer to 3.2 kcal per gram

If you are concerned about your protein intake, you can get all your daily requirements through a well-balanced, plant-based diet with sufficient calories. You will find plenty of delicious recipes in this book as well as a detailed nutrition guide.

CHAPTER 4:
PLANT-BASED BESTIES - THE PROTEIN SOURCES FOR MAXIMUM IMPACT

1. **Lentils** - Cooked lentils contain the following nutritional values per 125 grams:
    - Fat: 0.5 grams
    - Carbohydrates: 20 grams
    - Dietary fiber: 8 grams
    - Protein 9 grams

<u>The Health Benefits of Lentils</u>

Lentils are rich in polyphenols that protect the body against radiation, ultraviolet rays, heart disease, and cancer. They also help with weight maintenance and digestive health.

2. **Broccoli** - Raw broccoli contains the following nutritional values per 90 grams:
    - Fat: 0.3 grams
    - Carbohydrates: 6 grams
    - Dietary fiber: 2.4 grams
    - Protein: 2.6 grams

<u>The Health Benefits of Broccoli</u>

Broccoli contains several powerful nutrients such as vitamin K, which is essential for the blood clotting process, and vitamin C – a powerful antioxidant that protects the body against harmful free radicals.

3. **Nutritional Yeast** - Raw nutritional yeast contains the following nutritional values per 15 grams:

   - Fat: 0.5 grams
   - Carbohydrates: 5 grams
   - Dietary fiber: 3 grams
   - Protein: 8 grams

<u>The Health Benefits of Nutritional Yeast</u>

Nutritional yeast is high in vitamin B12, which helps to regulate the central nervous system, boosts energy, digestive system maintenance, protects the body against breast cancer, colon cancer, and stomach cancer. Nutritional yeast is good for people with diabetes because it contains no sugar and is therefore considered a low glycemic food.

4. **Peanut Butter Powder** - Raw peanut butter powder contains the following nutritional values per 13 grams:

   - Fat: 1.5 grams
   - Carbohydrates: 5 grams

- Dietary fiber: 1 gram
- Protein: 6 grams

The Health Benefits of Peanut Butter Powder

Peanut butter powder contains fewer calories and fat than regular peanut butter, making it beneficial for those wanting to reduce their fat and calorie intake. Peanut butter powder provides the same health benefits as peanut butter. It contains several nutrients that help to boost heart health, such as vitamin E, magnesium, polyunsaturated fatty acids, and monounsaturated fatty acids. It is a good source of magnesium, potassium, and iron, which improves blood circulation.

5. **Hemp Seeds** - Raw hemp seeds contain the following nutritional values per 28 grams:
   - Fat: 12 grams
   - Carbohydrates: 3 grams
   - Dietary fiber: 3 grams
   - Protein: 10 grams

The Health Benefits of Hemp Seeds

Hemp seeds are a powerful source of essential fatty acids, such as alpha-linolenic acid, which is an omega-3. They contain no trans fats, and they are low in unsaturated fats. Hemp seeds contain a wide range of vitamins and minerals, such as vitamin E, potassium, magnesium, and folate. They are high in omega-3 fatty acids, which improve heart health and reduce inflammation.

6. **Quinoa** - Raw quinoa contains the following nutritional values per 219 grams:

   - Fat: 2.4 grams
   - Carbohydrates: 25.7 grams
   - Dietary fiber: 2.8 grams
   - Protein: 5.7 grams

<u>The Health Benefits of Quinoa</u>

Quinoa contains almost double the amount of fiber than the majority of other grains. Fiber helps to reduce high blood pressure and therefore lower the risk of a heart attack. Quinoa is high in iron, which helps maintain the health of our red blood cells. Iron also boosts brain function because it helps carry oxygen to the brain. Quinoa is known to alleviate migraines because it assists in relaxing blood vessels.

7. **Sprouted Whole Grain Bread** - Raw sprouted whole grain bread contains the following nutritional values per slice (34 g):

   - Fat: 0.5 grams
   - Carbohydrates: 15 grams
   - Dietary fiber: 3 grams
   - Protein: 4 grams

<u>The Health Benefits of Whole Grain Bread</u>

Whole grains are packed with nutrients such as antioxidants, B vitamins, magnesium, copper, zinc, and iron. Studies have indicated that a diet rich in whole grains helps to reduce the risk of cancer, obesity, type 2 diabetes, and heart disease.

8. **Tofu** - Raw tofu contains the following nutritional values per 85 grams:
   - Fat: 3.5 grams
   - Carbohydrates: 2 grams
   - Dietary fiber: 1 gram
   - Protein: 8 grams

<u>The Health Benefits of Tofu</u>

Tofu is an excellent source of amino acids, calcium, iron, protein, and other micronutrients. Tofu comes from soy protein, which helps lower bad cholesterol. It is low in calories and gluten-free. It also contains isoflavones that protect the body against osteoporosis, heart disease, and cancer.

9. **Chia Seeds** - Dried chia seeds contain the following nutritional values for 28 grams:
   - Fat: 8.4 grams
   - Carbohydrates: 13 grams
   - Dietary fiber: 11 grams
   - Protein: 6 grams

<u>The Health Benefits of Chia Seeds</u>

Chia seeds are high in protein. One of the many benefits of protein is that it helps to control appetite, and therefore, plays a role in the weight loss process. Chia seeds are also rich in omega-3 fatty acids; the combination of omega-3's and protein stabilize blood sugar and improves metabolic health.

10. **Edamame Beans** - Raw edamame beans contain the following nutritional values per half a cup (75 g):

   - Fat: 5 grams
   - Carbohydrates: 9 grams
   - Dietary fiber: 8 grams
   - Protein: 12 grams

<u>The Health Benefits of Edamame Beans</u>

Edamame beans are high in protein and low in fat, and studies indicate that people who follow a high protein, low-fat diet achieve significant weight loss because they experience less hunger between meals.

11. **Tempeh** - Raw tempeh contains the following nutritional values per 84 grams:

   - Fat: 6 grams
   - Carbohydrates: 8 grams
   - Dietary fiber: 5 grams
   - Protein: 16 grams

The Health Benefits of Tempeh

Tempeh is a highly nutritious soy product that is high in protein, prebiotics, and a wide range of vitamins and minerals. Tempeh contains calcium, but it is dairy-free; since tempeh comes from soybeans, it contains isoflavones, which is a natural plant compound that helps reduce cholesterol levels.

12. **Chickpeas** - Raw chickpeas contains the following nutritional values per 82 grams:
    - Fat: 2 grams
    - Carbohydrates: 22 grams
    - Dietary fiber: 6 grams
    - Protein: 7 grams

The Health Benefits of Chickpeas

Chickpeas are low in calories and high in protein, which accelerates the weight loss process. They are also high in fiber, and the combination of protein and fiber assist in weight management because they suppress the appetite. Chickpeas are also considered a low glycemic food which is beneficial for blood sugar management.

13. **Peanuts** - Raw peanuts contain the following nutritional values per 32 grams:
    - Fat: 16 grams
    - Carbohydrates: 6 grams

- Dietary fiber: 2 grams
- Protein: 7 grams

The Health Benefits of Peanuts

Peanuts are low in carbohydrates and rich in nutrients; they contain polyunsaturated fats and monounsaturated fats. They help to improve blood cholesterol levels, which reduce the risk of stroke and heart disease. Peanuts are full of fiber and protein and help with weight maintenance. The bonus is that they also make a satisfying snack.

14. **Almonds** - Raw almonds contain the following nutritional values per 95 grams:
    - Fat: 47 grams
    - Carbohydrates: 21 grams
    - Dietary fiber: 12 grams
    - Protein: 20 grams

The Health Benefits of Almonds

Almonds are very nutritious and high in vitamins, minerals, antioxidants, and healthy fats. Almonds are rich in vitamin E, a fat-soluble antioxidant that protects the cells from oxidative stress. Several studies have linked vitamin E with lower rates of Alzheimer's disease, cancer, and heart disease.

15. **Spirulina** - Raw spirulina contains the following nutritional values per 10 grams:
- Fat: 0.8 grams
- Carbohydrates: 2.5 grams
- Dietary fiber: 0.4 grams
- Protein: 6 grams

The Health Benefits of Spirulina

Spirulina contains powerful antioxidants that protect the body against inflammation, cancer, and oxidative damage. It has a positive impact on cholesterol by lowering triglycerides and bad cholesterol at the same time as raising good cholesterol. Spirulina assists in lowering blood pressure, which helps to reduce the risk of conditions such as stroke and heart disease.

16. **Spelt** - Raw spelt contains the following nutritional values per 100 grams:
- Fat: 2.4 grams
- Carbohydrates: 70 grams
- Dietary fiber: 11 grams
- Protein: 15 grams

The Health Benefits of Spelt

Spelt is rich in many nutrients such as niacin, zinc, potassium, magnesium, and iron. It is known to help reduce the cholesterol absorbed into the bloodstream. Additionally, the high fiber content in spelt helps reduce blood pressure. They lower the risk of stroke and heart disease.

17. **Potatoes** - Raw potatoes contain the following nutritional values per 1 potato (148 grams):

- Fat: 0 grams
- Carbohydrates: 26 grams
- Dietary fiber: 2 grams
- Protein: 3 grams

The Health Benefits of Potatoes

Potatoes are high in compounds such as phenolic acids, carotenoids, and flavonoids. They play the same role as antioxidants and protect the body against free radicals, thereby reducing the risk of chronic conditions such as cancer, diabetes, and heart disease. The resistant starch in potatoes also helps to improve digestive health.

18. **Kale** - Raw kale contains the following nutritional values per cup:
- Fat: 0.1 grams
- Carbohydrates: 1.4 grams
- Dietary fiber: 0.6 grams
- Protein: 0.7 grams

The Health Benefits of Kale

Kale is one of the most nutritious plants in the world, and it contains 4.5 times more vitamin C than spinach. Vitamin C is an important water-soluble antioxidant required for essential cell functions. Kale is also one of the world's best sources of vitamin K, which is crucial for blood clotting.

19. **Mushrooms** - Raw mushrooms contain the following nutritional values per half a cup (48 grams):

- Fat: 0 grams
- Carbohydrates: 2 grams
- Dietary fiber: 1 gram
- Protein: 1 gram

The Health Benefits of Mushrooms

Mushrooms are an excellent source of folic acid. They are said to help boost the health of babies while in the womb. They are also high in selenium, and studies suggest they protect against cognitive decline, thyroid disease, heart disease, and cancer.

20. **Seitan**: Raw seitan contain the following nutritional values per 100 grams:
- Fat: 1.9 grams
- Carbohydrates: 14 grams

- Dietary fiber: 0.6 grams
- Protein: 75 grams

<u>The Health Benefits of Seitan</u>

Seitan is a good source of protein, and it is low in calories; it is one of the few meat substitutes that doesn't contain soy. Seitan is high in iron, which increases energy and enhances athletic performance.

CHAPTER 5:
THE ROLE OF MICRONUTRIENTS AND FOOD SUPPLEMENTS

Micronutrients refer to vitamins and minerals; the body does not need as many micronutrients as it does macronutrients, hence the name. Despite this, the body does not produce vitamins and minerals, we can only access them through food.

Vitamins and Minerals

All vitamins and minerals are found in healthy foods; therefore, you will not need to take vitamin and mineral supplements if your diet and caloric intake is sufficient and includes a wide range of whole foods. There is no standard requirement for vitamin and mineral intake, as this varies with age, gender, and several other factors.

Before taking any supplements, a blood test is advisable to determine whether you need to boost your vitamin and mineral intake. It is also helpful to have blood tests periodically to ensure you are not suffering from any deficiencies.

There may be times when your vitamin intake is better than others. For example, during the summer months, high levels of vitamin D can be found in the body. During the winter, it has the potential to drop below a healthy level; in which case, you will require vitamin D supplements.

Vegetarians and vegans are prone to the following vitamin and mineral deficiencies:

- Vitamin B12
- Vitamin D
- Calcium
- Iron

These vitamins are present in the following plant-based sources:

- Calcium: Leafy green vegetables such as kale and spinach, sesame seeds, almonds, and calcium-fortified milk and yogurt alternatives.
- Iron: Leafy green vegetables such as kale and spinach, pumpkin seeds, quinoa, and legumes.
- Vitamin B12: Nutritional yeast.
- Vitamin D: Mushrooms, GHT, and Source of life supplements for vegans.

As mentioned, all the required vitamins and minerals are available in whole foods. However, because vitamin B12 is not available in vegan whole foods, there is some debate surrounding whether there is sufficient availability in breakfast cereals, fortified plant milk, and yeast extract. Therefore, to avoid a deficiency, it is advised that those on a plant-based diet take a daily supplement.

CHAPTER 6:
BULKING AND CUTTING - A QUICK & EFFECTIVE STEP-BY-STEP GUIDE

Weight loss requires burning more calories than you consume; this doesn't sound too difficult. However, everyday distractions can often get in the way of our ability to effectively monitor our food intake. One way to overcome this problem is through calorie counting; people often use this strategy when trying to lose weight.

Calories – What Are They?

Calories determine the amount of energy present in food and drink. The body needs energy to perform essential functions such as thinking, breathing, and walking. We put on weight when we don't use the calories we consume because any leftovers are stored as fat.

Calorie Counting – What's the Point?

You will often hear that it isn't necessary to count calories for weight loss, but several studies have proved otherwise. These studies involve getting participants to eat excess amounts of food to measure how it affects their health and weight. All the results from these studies have drawn the same conclusions: weight gain is caused by eating more calories than you burn. The findings prove that weight loss is possible for those who can commit to reducing their calorie intake.

Calorie Intake – How Many?

Several factors determine how many calories you should consume: these include weight, age, gender, and activity level. Use an online calorie counting calculator that will help you determine how many calories you should consume.

Calorie Counting App

The good news is that calorie-counting apps have simplified the process making it easy for you to count your calories throughout the day. Here are some of the most popular calorie counting apps:

- My Fitness Pal
- Cron-o-meter
- SparkPeople
- Lose It!
- FatSecret

Calorie Counting Does Not Justify Unhealthy Eating

When it comes to health and weight loss, what you eat is more important than the calories you count. So, if you eat French fries worth 100 calories and broccoli worth 100 calories, the calories you consume from these two foods are not of equal value. It is also important to mention that the type of food you eat will also affect your appetite, hormones, hunger levels, and the number of calories you burn.

If you want to lose weight and remain healthy, most nutritionists recommend that you stick to a plant-based diet containing high-quality unprocessed foods.

Calorie Counting Success Tips

- Get Ready: Download one of the calorie-counting apps or use one of the websites.
- Create a meal plan and work out how you are going to estimate or measure your portions.
- Pay Attention to Food Labels: When it comes to calorie counting, food labels are very helpful. They also give you the recommended portion sizes for meals.
- Eliminate Temptation: Keep healthy snacks at home and get rid of any junk food.

- Don't Try and Lose Weight Too Fast: One of the mistakes that people make during the weight loss process is they try and lose weight too fast. The quickest way to put weight back on after losing it is to lose weight too quickly.

What is Basal Metabolic Rate?

Also referred to as BMR, the basal metabolic rate is the energy your body burns when it is resting each day. Put another way, it is the amount of energy your body needs to continue functioning while you are taking a break from physical activities.

The body always needs energy even when you are asleep because it never stops functioning. Your heart is still beating; your body is still digesting food; your brain is still in operation, etc. In order for the body to function effectively, it must use approximately 70 percent of the calories you consume.

Your BMR also affects weight loss, and the more muscle mass you have, the better your BMR. Extra muscles help calories burn faster, which causes a decrease in body fat. If you are planning on going on a diet program, you can use your BMR as a baseline. Depending on your activity level, you can add extra calories. The more physically active you are, the more calories you will burn, and the more muscles you will build. Therefore, to keep your body fit and healthy, you will need to pay attention to the calories you consume.

Metabolic rate changes with age. BMR peaks between the ages of 16-17 and starts decreasing after this. A low BMR will require you to consume fewer calories to lose body fat. You can work out your metabolic age by comparing your BMR to the average BMR of your age group. If you have a higher metabolic rate than your age, it's an indication that you need to improve your metabolic rate. High-intensity workouts will build healthy muscle tissue, and this will improve your metabolic age. You will know when you need to gain more muscle mass if you keep track of your metabolic age.

What is Total Daily Energy Expenditure?
Total daily energy expenditure (TDEE) is the total number of calories you burn in a day. Four main factors determine it:

- Basal metabolic rate
- Thermic effect of activity
- Non-exercise activity thermogenesis
- Thermic effect of food

We have already discussed the basal metabolic rate so we will focus on the other three factors:

Thermic effect of activity (TEA): Refers to the number of calories burned due to exercise. Not only does TEA vary between one person to another, but for the same person, it can vary from day-to-day. The length of the workout, the frequency of training and the intensity of training all affect your TEA.

Non-exercise activity thermogenesis (NEAT): Makes up the number of calories used during the day from physical activity that isn't exercising. NEAT can include things like walking up the stairs, moving from one room to the next, or walking the dog, etc. NEAT varies between people, and it can have either a small or large impact on your overall TDEE, depending on how physically active you are during the day. For example, a construction worker or a waitress is going to have a significantly higher NEAT than someone who works from home and spends all day sitting at their desk.

Thermic effect of food (TFE): The digestion process requires energy. TFE stands for the thermic effect of food, and it involves breaking down the fat, carbohydrates, and protein you consume into fatty acids, sugars, and amino acids that are then absorbed by the body and used to perform functions such as producing neurotransmitters, synthesizing hormones, and developing new tissues. Research suggests that the TFE typically accounts for 10 percent of your total daily energy expenditure. But depending on the exact macronutrient composition of your diet, it can either be slightly higher or lower. For example, it takes more energy to digest protein than it does fat or carbohydrates. Therefore, you are going to burn more calories if you are eating a high protein diet than if you ate the same number of calories on a low protein diet.

Your TDEE is the total of the above factors when you add up all these numbers. You get an estimate of the number of calories you need to consume each day to maintain your current weight. However, you can make the process of calculating your TDEE easier with an online calculator.

What is Your Goal?

What do you aim to achieve? Do you want to bulk up (gain weight) or cut (lose weight)? The following figures provide you with a simple way of matching what you want to achieve with a value:

- For weight loss, you will require a – 20% drop
- For slow weight loss, you will expect a – 10% drop
- To maintain your weight, 0%
- To gain weight slowly, you will need + 10%
- To gain weight, you will need + 20%

The number is an indication of the caloric deficit or surplus. For example, +20 % means that your daily goal for your calorie intake should be 20 % higher than your TDEE.

Macronutrient Calorie Density

- Carbohydrates: 4 calories per gram
- Protein: 4 calories per gram
- Fat: 9 calories per gram

You can start working on your goal by determining how much protein you will need to consume. You will find everything you need to know in chapter 3. The remainder of your calories will be split into fats and carbohydrates.

Carbohydrates - Fat Calorie Split

After you have worked out your protein consumption, the next stage is determining how many calories you will need to split between fats and carbohydrates. There is no standard amount; it will depend on your personal preference. Your body might respond better to more fats and fewer carbs, or vice versa. There is a higher chance that you will prefer more carbohydrates if you are more physically active.

A rule that people typically follow is not to consume anything less than 0.25 grams of fat per pound. Even though this seems like a pretty easy target, when you are on a hard cut, and you are not working with that many calories, it can be difficult to stick to. Over a long period of time, anything less than this amount of fat can lead to issues such as dry hair and skin and other health issues.

Counting Example

Below is an example of how you can calculate macronutrients for a 2,000-calorie diet made up of 40% carbohydrates, 30% protein, and 30% fat.

Carbohydrates:
- Per gram – 4 calories
- 40% of 2,000 calories = 800 calories from carbohydrates per day
- Total grams of carbohydrates allowed per day = 800/4 = 200 grams

Fats:

- Per gram – 9 calories
- 30% of 2,000 calories – 600 calories of fats per day
- Total grams of fat allowed per day = 600/9 = 67 grams

Proteins:

- Per gram – 4 calories
- 30% of 2,000 calories – 600 calories of protein per day
- Total grams of fat allowed per day = 600/4 = 150 grams

In this case, your recommended daily intake would be 67 grams of fat, 150 grams of protein, and 200 grams of carbohydrates.

Now that you have a full understanding of the basics of sports nutrition, it's time to try out some delicious recipes so that you can really get to experience the full benefits of a plant-based diet!

CHAPTER 7:
GOOD MORNING, SUNSHINE! QUICK MEALS TO POWER YOUR DAY

PECAN-MAPLE GRANOLA

Cooking Time: 25 Minute - Servings: 4 Servings
Calories: 220/Protein: 5 grams/Fat: 7 grams/Carbs: 35
grams/Fiber: 4 grams

Make your own healthy and delicious granola in less than half an hour. The two main ingredients in this recipe are rolled oats and pecan pieces. Rolled oats are high in soluble fiber which helps lower glucose and cholesterol levels. Pecans are a good source of monounsaturated fats which support heart health by lowering bad cholesterol levels.

Ingredients

- 1 teaspoon of vanilla extract
- ¼ cup of maple syrup
- ¼ cup of pecan pieces
- 1 ½ cups of rolled oats
- ½ a teaspoon of ground cinnamon
- Non-dairy milk of your choice

Directions

1. Prepare the oven by heating it to 300 degrees F.
2. Place parchment paper over a baking tray.

3. Combine the cinnamon, vanilla, maple syrup, pecan pieces and oats in a large bowl and stir to combine.
4. Transfer the mixture onto the baking tray and spread it over evenly.
5. Bake for 20 minutes, shift the granola around after 10 minutes.
6. Once cooked, take the granola out of the oven and leave it to cool down for 30 minutes.
7. Store in a container and serve with non-dairy milk.

BREAKFAST SCRAMBLE

Cooking Time: 20 Minute - Servings: 2 Servings
Calories: 230/Protein: 27 grams/Fat: 10 grams/Carbs: 16
grams/Fiber: 7 grams

This delicious scramble makes a satisfying side dish or a main breakfast dish. The two main ingredients in this recipe are tofu and mushrooms. Tofu is valuable plant source of calcium which is an important mineral required for bone health. Mushrooms are high in vitamin B which is responsible for keeping the cells healthy and boosting energy levels.

Ingredients

- 1 cup of fresh spinach
- 1/8 teaspoon of black pepper
- ½ a teaspoon of onion powder
- ½ teaspoon of garlic powder
- 1 tablespoon of vegetable broth
- 2 tablespoons of nutritional yeast
- ½ a diced bell pepper
- 4 ounces of sliced mushrooms
- 1 packet of extra firm tofu

Directions

1. Over medium temperature, heat a large frying pan.

2. Drain the tofu, place it in a bowl and mash it down with a fork.

3. Transfer the tofu into the frying pan and add the, pepper, garlic powder, onion powder, broth, nutritional yeast, bell pepper and mushrooms. Put a lid on the frying pan and leave it to cook for 10 minutes. Stir the ingredients after 5 minutes.

4. Add the spinach and cook for another 5 minutes, divide onto plates and serve.

LOADED BREAKFAST BURRITO

Cooking Time: 25 Minutes - Servings: 2 Servings
Calories: 535/Protein: 29 grams/Fat: 8 grams/Carbs: 95 grams/Fiber: 21 grams

Kick start your day with this scrumptious plant powered nutritious burrito! The two main ingredients in this recipe are tofu and black beans. Tofu is a good plant source of iron which plays an important role in the immune function. Black beans are rich in copper is required to help maintain healthy nerves, blood vessels and bones.

Ingredients

- 6 corn tortillas
- ¼ cup of salsa
- ½ a teaspoon of onion powder
- ½ a teaspoon of garlic powder
- 1 tablespoon of nutritional yeast
- 2 tablespoons of vegetable broth
- 1 diced and seeded jalapeno
- 4 ounces of sliced mushrooms
- 1 cup of cooked blacked beans
- 2 diced medium potatoes
- ½ a block of firm tofu

Directions

1. Prepare the oven by heating it to 300 degrees F.
2. Line a baking tray with parchment paper.
3. Over medium-low temperature, heat a frying pan.
4. Drain the tofu, place it in a bowl and mash it up with a fork.
5. Transfer the tofu into the frying pan.
6. Add the onion powder, garlic powder, nutritional yeast, broth, jalapeno, mushrooms, black beans and potatoes, stir to combine.
7. Turn the heat down to low, put a lid on the frying pan and leave the ingredients to cook for 10 minutes.
8. Add the salsa, stir to combine and cook for a further 5 minutes.
9. Put the tortillas on the baking tray and heat for 30 seconds.
10. Remove the tortillas from the oven and lay them onto plates. Fill the burritos with filling, roll them up and serve.

FRUITY OATMEAL

Cooking Time: 25 Minutes - Servings: 2 Servings
Calories: 230/Protein: 4.6 grams/Fat: 5.6 grams/Carbs:
43.8 grams

This satisfying and nutrient dense oatmeal will fire up your day and get you ready give you everything you need to get going. Two of the main ingredients are apples and prunes. Apples are high in fiber and water which help you to feel full and satisfied. Prunes are a powerful source of the mineral boron, which help to build strong muscles and bones.

Ingredients

- ½ a cup of fresh and frozen apple juice
- ½ a cup of oatmeal
- ½ a cup of water
- 3 diced prunes
- 1 small, diced apple
- 4 diced pecans
- 3 dried and diced, dehydrated apricots
- ¼ teaspoon of cinnamon

Directions

1. In a small saucepan combine the water and apple juice and bring the mixture to a boil.

2. Add the oatmeal, stir to combine and leave it to cook for one minute.
3. Add the fruit pieces, cinnamon and pecans, stir to combine.
4. Pour into bowls and serve.

BREAKFAST CEREAL

Cooking Time: 45 Minutes - Servings: 6 Servings
Calories: 160/Protein: 3 grams/Fat: 1.5 grams/Carbs: 34
grams

A delicious plant-based breakfast cereal that is simple to make and much healthier than store bought brands. Two of the main ingredients are brown rice and raisins. Brown rice is high in flavonoids and phenols, a class of antioxidants that assist in protecting the body against oxidative stress. Half a cup of raisins contains 45 milligrams of calcium which is approximately 4 percent of your daily requirement. Calcium is essential for healthy teeth and bones.

Ingredients
- ¼ tablespoon of butter
- 2 ¼ cups of water
- Honey
- 1 teaspoon of cinnamon
- 1 cup of uncooked brown rice
- ½ a cup of seedless raisins

Directions

1. Combine the butter, rice, raisins and cinnamon in a saucepan, add the water and bring the ingredients to a boil. Cover and leave to simmer for 40 minutes and fluff with a fork.
2. Pour into bowls and serve with honey as a sweetener.

VEGETABLE HASH

*Cooking Time: 35 Minutes - Servings: 4 Servings
Calories: 273/Protein: 9 grams/Fat: 11 grams/Carbs: 39
grams*

This delightful medley of vegetables is packed with peppers, garlic, onions and black beans. It's affordable, versatile and ready to eat in less than an hour. Two of the main ingredients are Swiss chard and tomatoes. Swiss chard is an excellent source of vitamin K which is essential for bone health and important functions in the body such as blood clotting.

Ingredients

- 1 tablespoon of chopped sage leaves
- 1 diced bell pepper
- 3 cloves of minced garlic
- 1 diced onion
- 3 tablespoons of olive oil
- 3 diced red tomatoes
- 1 can of 15-ounce black beans
- 1 tablespoon of chopped parsley
- 2 cups of chopped swiss chard
- Sea salt and black pepper

Direction

1. Cook the onion, garlic, and potato in a skillet with oil, this should take approximately 20 minutes.
2. Add the swiss chard and the beans and cook for a further three minutes.
3. Serve with parsley and season with salt and pepper.

CHOCOLATE & QUINOA BOWL

Cooking Time: 35 Minutes - Servings: 2 Servings
Calories: 392/Protein: 12 grams/Fat: 19 grams/Carbs: 49
grams

The mouthwatering breakfast really does put the 'good' in your morning! The chocolate flavor in this bowl makes it completely irresistible! Two of the main ingredients are banana and almond butter. Banana is an instant energy booster containing a powerhouse of nutrients such as folate, iron, magnesium and calcium. Banana is known as a brain food because of its high potassium content which helps to keep you alert. Almond butter is an excellent source of monounsaturated fats which helps to keep the heart healthy.

Ingredients

- 1 cup of quinoa
- 1 cup of unsweetened almond milk
- 1 teaspoon of cinnamon
- 1 cup of water
- 1 banana
- ¼ cup of fresh raspberries
- 2 tablespoons of walnuts (optional)
- 2 tablespoons of almond butter
- 2-3 tablespoons of unsweetened cocoa powder

Directions

1. Combine the quinoa, water, milk and cinnamon in a saucepan and bring the ingredients to a boil. Turn the heat down to low and allow it to simmer for twenty minutes.
2. Puree the banana, add the cocoa powder, flaxseed and almond butter and stir to combine.
3. Pour into bowls and top with walnuts (if you want) and pudding and serve.

MANGO SMOOTHIE

Cooking Time: 5 Minutes - Servings: 3 Servings
Calories: 376/Protein: 5 grams/Fat: 2 grams/Carbs: 95
grams

This super creamy mango smoothie is great for those mornings when you are pushed for time, not only does it taste amazing, it only takes 5 minutes to make. Two of the main ingredients are mango and peaches. Mango skin contains phytochemicals which acts as natural fat busters. Peaches are high in the trace element zinc which is required for a healthy immune system.

Ingredients

- 1 peeled and chopped carrot
- 1 cup of strawberries
- 1 cup of water
- 1 cup of chopped peaches
- 1 sliced frozen banana
- 1 cup of chopped mango

Directions

1. Combine all the ingredients in a food processor, blend until smooth and serve.

FRUIT SALAD

*Cooking Time: 15 Minutes - Servings: 4 Servings
Calories: 276/Protein: 3.1 grams/Fat: 12.3 grams/Carbs:
39.7 grams*

Wake up to this incredibly refreshing and tasty fruit salad, what better way to start your day than with a bowl of delicious, fresh fruit bursting with flavor. Two of the main ingredients in this recipe are pineapples and oranges. Pineapples contain bromelain which is an inflammatory property that reduces the time it takes to recover after a workout.

Ingredients

- 1/8 teaspoon of cinnamon
- 1/8 teaspoon of ginger
- 1/8 teaspoon of cardamom
- 1 tablespoon of lime, juiced and zest
- 1 cup of ripe mango, peeled and diced
- 1 cup of orange sections
- 1 cup of sliced banana
- 2 cups of cubed fresh pineapple
- 1 tablespoon of vegan dark brown sugar (optional)

Directions

1. Combine all the ingredients together in a bowl and refrigerate for an hour before serving.

HASH BROWNS WITH EGG PLANT

Cooking Time: 20 Minutes - Servings: 8 Servings
Calories: 100/Protein: 2.42 grams/Fat: 6.4 grams/Carbs: 8
grams

A luscious, low-carb, easy to make breakfast that the whole family will love. Two of the main ingredients in this recipe are eggplant and bell peppers. Eggplants are rich in phytonutrients which increases blood flow to the brain making you more alert. Red bell peppers contain more than 200 percent of your daily vitamin C intake. Vitamin C is a powerful antioxidant that boosts the immune system.

Ingredients

- 1 peeled, salted and cubed eggplant
- 2 tablespoons of coconut oil
- 1 diced red onion
- Sea salt and pepper
- ½ a teaspoon of cinnamon
- ¼ teaspoon of cayenne pepper
- ½ a teaspoon of coriander seeds
- ½ a cup of chopped and drained sundried tomatoes
- ¼ cup of fresh mint leaves
- ¼ cup of toasted and slivered almonds

- 4 cloves of minced garlic
- 2 red bell peppers, diced and seeded

Ingredients

1. Heat the oil in a frying pan, sear the eggplant and bell pepper and cook for three minutes, stir occasionally.
2. Add the garlic and onion and cook for a further two minutes.
3. Add the tomatoes, almonds and mint leaves, make sure it heated all the way through and then add the rest of the ingredients.
4. Divide onto plates and serve.

CHIA, PUMPKIN SMOOTHIE

*Cooking Time: 5 Minutes - Servings: 1 Serving
Calories: 726/Protein: 5.5 grams/Fat: 69.8 grams/Carbs: 15
grams*

Rise and shine! This healthy, delectable pumpkin smoothie is exactly what you need to put some pep in your step the first thing in the morning. Two of the main ingredients in this recipe are avocado and pumpkin spice. Avocado contain zeaxanthin and lutein, two phytochemicals that protect the eyes against ultraviolet light. Pumpkin spice contains cinnamon which is an excellent anti-inflammatory that relieves muscle stiffness and pain.

Ingredients

- ½ a teaspoon of pumpkin pie spice
- 1 teaspoon of pure vanilla
- ½ a fresh avocado
- ¾ cup of full fat coconut milk

Directions

1. Combine all the ingredients in a food processor, and blend until smooth.

FLAXSEED PANCAKES

*Cooking Time: 15 Minutes - Servings: 1 Serving
Calories: 309/Protein: 13.4 grams/Fat: 27.1 grams/Carbs: 5
grams*

For those lazy mornings why not indulge in low-carb yummy flaxseed pancake? Two of the main ingredients are flaxseeds and coconut oil. Flaxseeds are a popular superfood with many health benefits, they are high in omega-3 fatty acids which lowers the risk of heart disease. Coconut oil is high in medium chain fatty acids which boost energy and endurance.

Ingredients

- 3 tablespoons of water
- ¼ teaspoon of baking powder
- ½ scoop of vanilla vegan powder
- 1 ½ teaspoons of coconut oil
- A pinch of sea salt
- 2 tablespoons of flaxseeds

Directions

1. In a small bowl, combine one tablespoon of flaxseed and water and stir to combine.
2. Add the oil and stir to combine.

3. In a separate bowl, add the rest of the flaxseed, protein powder, baking powder and salt, stir to combine.
4. Pour the dry ingredients into the wet ingredients and stir to combine.
5. Heat a non-stick frying pan over a medium temperature.
6. Pour the batter out into the pan and let it cook for five minutes, flip the pancake and cook for a further two minutes.
7. Repeat until the batter is finished, arrange on a plate and serve.

AVOCADO BREAKFAST BOWL

Cooking Time: 5 Minutes - Servings: 1 Serving
Calories: 562/Protein: 8 grams/Fat: 52 grams/Carbs: 7
grams

Wake up to a mouth-watering assortment of avocado, ginger, tahini and much more. Two of the main ingredients in this recipe are avocado and carrots. Avocado are high in polyunsaturated fats which are essential for muscle movement. Carrots are an excellent source of beta carotene which is a powerful antioxidant that protects the body against free radicals.

Ingredients for the Sauce

- 1/4 cup of lemon juice
- 1 tablespoon of poppy seeds
- 1 tablespoon of grated, fresh ginger
- ¼ cup of olive oil
- Sea salt

Ingredients for the Avocado

- 1 avocado, pit removed and halved
- 1 shredded carrot
- 2 tablespoons of Tahini

Directions

1. In a small bowl, whisk together all the ingredients for the sauce.
2. Arrange the avocado ingredients on a plate drizzle the sauce over the top.

STRAWBERRY COCONUT BARS

Cooking Time: 4 hours 10 Minutes - Servings: 2 Servings Calories: 294/Protein: 3 grams/Fat: 28 grams/Carbs: 4 grams

These dreamy strawberry coconut bars will have you flying out of bed in the morning in anticipation of these yummy treats. Two of the main ingredients are strawberries and coconut. Strawberries are an excellent source of vitamin K which supports the maintenance of strong bones. Coconuts are high in potassium which help regulate blood pressure and balance sodium levels in the body.

Ingredients

- 1 tablespoon of coconut oil
- ¼ cup of unsweetened coconut flakes
- 1 teaspoon of Stevia
- 16 ounces of melted coconut butter
- 1 cup of chopped strawberries

Directions

1. In a small bowl, combine the butter, oil and stevia, stir to combine and then transfer the mixture into a baking dish.
2. Add the coconut and the strawberries, stir to combine and leave in the fridge for four hours.
3. Once firm, chop into bars and serve.

BLUEBERRY AND FLAXSEED OATMEAL

Cooking Time: 15 Minutes - Servings: 2 Servings
Calories: 430/Protein: 10 grams/Fat: 34 grams/Carbs: 12
grams

This wholesome bowl of blueberry and flaxseed oatmeal makes for a very tasty treat first thing in the morning. The two main ingredients in this recipe are blueberries and flaxseed. Blueberries are high in magnesium, calcium and potassium which help to reduce blood pressure. Flaxseeds are high in fiber which helps lower cholesterol and regulate blood sugar.

Ingredients

- 10 drops of stevia
- 1 teaspoon of vanilla extract
- A pinch of sea salt
- ¼ cup of ground flaxseed
- ¼ cup of coconut flour
- 1 cup of almond milk

Ingredients for Garnish

- 2 ounces of blueberries
- 2 tablespoons of almond butter
- 2 tablespoons of pumpkin seeds
- 1 ounce if shaved coconut

Directions

1. Heat the almond milk over a low temperature in a saucepan.
2. Add the flaxseed, cinnamon, salt and coconut flour and stir to combine.
3. When the ingredients start to bubble, add the stevia and vanilla.
4. Pour into bowls, garnish and serve.

CHAPTER 8:
LUNCHTIME - STAPLE MEALS
TO GET YOU THROUGH THE DAY

SAUTÉED COLLARD GREENS

*Cooking Time: 35 Minutes - Servings: 4 Servings
Calories: 28/Protein: 3 grams/Fat: 1 grams/Carbs: 4
grams/Fiber: 2 grams*

A simple and delicious nutrient dense meal for the perfect lunch. The two main ingredients in this recipe are collard greens and garlic powder. Collard greens are a rich source of vitamin K which is a fat-soluble vitamin that plays a role in blood clotting. Garlic is known for its antibiotic properties; it is also good for gut health.

Ingredients

- 1/8 teaspoon of black pepper
- ½ a teaspoon of onion powder
- ½ a teaspoon of garlic powder
- 1 cup of vegetable broth
- 1 ½ pounds of collard greens

Directions

1. Separate the hard-middle stems from the greens, and roughly chop the leaves.
2. Combine the vegetable broth, pepper, onion powder and garlic powder in a saucepan and bring it to a boil. Add the greens, put a lid on

the saucepan, turn the heat down to low and leave the ingredients to cook for 20 minutes. Stir every five minutes.

3. Divide into bowls and serve.

CRISPY CAULIFLOWER WINGS

*Cooking Time: 50 Minutes - Servings: 6 Servings
Calories: 96/Protein: 3 grams/Fat: 1 grams/Carbs: 20
grams/Fiber: 2 grams*

These crispy cauliflower wings are equally as delicious but much healthier than chicken wings. The main ingredients in this recipe are cauliflower and onion powder. Cauliflower is high in fiber which helps maintain bowel health. Onions are an excellent source of antioxidants that reduce cholesterol levels and fight inflammation.

Ingredients

- 1 head of cauliflower, chopped into bite sized florets
- ¼ teaspoon of freshly ground black pepper
- ½ a teaspoon of paprika
- 2 teaspoons of onion powder
- 2 teaspoons of garlic powder
- ¾ cup of whole-wheat flour
- 1 cup of oat milk

Directions

1. Prepare the oven by preheating it to 425 degrees F.
2. Lay parchment paper over a baking tray.

3. Combine the pepper, paprika, onion powder, garlic powder, flour and milk in a large bowl and whisk to combine.

4. Add the cauliflower florets to the bowl and toss to coat.

5. Arrange the florets onto the baking tray and bake for 40 minutes until they become crispy and turn into a golden-brown color. Turn the cauliflower after 20 minutes.

6. Remove the cauliflower wings from the oven and serve.

MASHED POTATOES WITH GRAVY

Cooking Time: 25 Minutes - Servings: 6 Servings
Calories: 260/Protein: 8 grams/Fat: 1 grams/Carbs: 56
grams/Fiber: 4 grams

Delicious creamy mashed potatoes with gravy for a satisfying lunch to keep you full until dinner time. The two main ingredients in this recipe are potatoes and thyme. Potatoes are a rich source of folate which the body needs to convert carbohydrates into energy. Thyme is an excellent source of vitamin A which supports a healthy immune system.

Ingredients for the Mashed Potatoes
- 1 teaspoon of onion powder
- 1 teaspoon of garlic powder
- ½ a cup of plant-based milk
- 8 red potatoes sliced into cubes

The Ingredients for the Gravy
- ¼ teaspoon of dried sage
  ¼ teaspoon of dried thyme
- ¼ teaspoon of black pepper
- ½ teaspoon of onion powder
- ½ a teaspoon of garlic powder
- ¼ cup of gluten-free flour
- 2 cups of vegetable broth, divided

Directions for the Mashed Potatoes

1. Boil a large saucepan full of water on high heat and add the potatoes. Put a lid on the saucepan, turn the heat down to a medium temperature and boil for 15 minutes, the potatoes are ready when you can easily pierce them with a fork.

2. Pour the liquid out and put the potatoes back into the saucepan.

3. Use a potato masher to mash the potatoes until they become smooth.

4. Add the onion powder, garlic powder and milk and stir to combine.

Directions to Make the Gravy

1. In a medium sized saucepan, combine the flour and half a cup of broth and whisk together thoroughly. Add the rest of the broth and stir to combine.

2. Add the sage, thyme, pepper, onion powder and garlic powder and stir to combine while it's on medium heat. Reduce the temperature to low and leave the ingredients to simmer for 10 minutes.

3. Divide the mashed potatoes onto plates, pour the gravy over the top and serve.

MEDITERRANEAN WRAP

*Cooking Time: 10 Minutes - Servings: 1 Serving
Calories: 428/Protein: 13 grams/Fat: 23 grams/Carbs: 47
grams*

These plant-based Mediterranean wraps feature crispy chickpeas, juicy olives and succulent cherry tomatoes. They are quick and easy to make for a great snack on the go or a packed lunch. The two main ingredients in this recipe are chickpeas and spinach. Chickpeas are high in the soluble fiber raffinose which is a good bacteria that promotes colon health. Spinach is high in iron which assists in carrying oxygen around the body.

Ingredients

- ¼ cup of crispy chickpeas
- ¼ cup of halved cherry tomatoes
- A handful of baby spinach
- 2 tablespoons of quartered kalamata olives
- ¼ cup of hummus
- 2 tablespoons of fresh lemon juice
- 2 Romaine lettuce leaves

Directions

1. In a small bowl, combine the lemon juice, kalamata olives, baby spinach, cherry tomatoes and chickpeas.

2. Spread the hummus over the lettuce leaves, top with the chickpea mixture, wrap and serve.

RED LENTIL SOUP

Cooking Time: 50 Minutes - Servings: 4 Servings
Calories: 188/Protein: 12.5 grams/Fat: 1.2 grams/Carbs:
33.6 grams

A scrumptious spicy blend of lentils paprika and onion. Two of the main ingredients in this recipe are red lentils and potatoes. Red lentils are a plentiful source of potassium, folic acid and fiber, all of which help to support heart health. Potatoes are an excellent source of zinc, magnesium and calcium, they all help to maintain and build bone strength and structure.

Ingredients

- 1 teaspoon of paprika
- 4 cups of vegetable stock
- ¼ cup of finely chopped onion
- 1 cup of red lentils
- ½ a cup of peeled and diced potato
- Sea salt and black pepper

Directions

1. Put the lentils into a medium sized saucepan and rinse them under cold water.
2. Add the paprika, onion, stock and potatoes to the pot and bring the ingredients to a boil.

Turn the heat down to a low temperature and leave it to simmer.

3. Place a lid on the saucepan and cook the ingredients until the lentils become tender. This will take around 30 minutes.

4. Add the salt and pepper, pour the soup into a food processor and blend until smooth.

5. Pour into bowls and serve.

MACARONI AND CHEESE

Cooking Time: 1 Hour 30 Minutes - Servings: 6 Servings Calories: 848/Protein: 70 grams/Fat: 8.4 grams/Carbs: 140.1 grams

Who said eating a plant-based diet was boring? This delicious macaroni and cheese are made up of a creamy sauce with a delicious crunchy topping. The main ingredients in this recipe are nutritional yeast and whole wheat bread. Nutritional yeast is a rich source of vitamin B12 which improves memory, boosts mood and prevents heart disease.

Ingredients

- Whole wheat breadcrumbs
- 3 cups of nutritional yeast
- 16 ounces of vegan mayonnaise
- 16 ounces of whole wheat elbow macaroni
- Milk substitute

Directions

1. Preheat the oven to 350 degrees F.
2. Cook the macaroni according to the directions on the packet.
3. Drain the water from the macaroni and add the vegan mayonnaise, nutritional yeast and stir to combine.

4. Add the milk substitute and keep stirring until it becomes creamy.
5. Pour the ingredients into a baking dish and sprinkle the whole wheat breadcrumbs over the top.
6. Bake for approximately 1 hour until it turns golden brown in color.

BLACK EYED PEAS STEW

Cooking Time: 30 Minutes - Servings: 5 Servings
Calories: 338/Protein: 21 grams/Fat: 4 grams/Carbs: 58
grams

Classic black-eyed peas are stewed with garlic pepper, tomatoes and okra. The two main ingredients in this recipe are black eyed peas and okra. Black eyed peas are low in fat and calories which help to maintain weight loss. Okra contains mucilage which is prevents cholesterol from being absorbed by the stools.

Ingredients

- 8 ounces of okra
- 2 cans of drained black-eyed peas
- 1 onion
- 2 tablespoons of olive oil
- 1 clove of garlic
- ¼ teaspoon of cayenne pepper
- 1 can of crushed tomatoes

Directions

1. Heat the olive oil in a frying pan and brown the onions.
2. Add the cayenne pepper and garlic, stir and cook for one minute.
3. Add the remaining ingredients and leave them to simmer until the okra becomes soft.

FALAFEL WRAP

Cooking Time: 1 Hour - Servings: 6 Servings
Calories: 546/Protein: 18 grams/Fat: 19 grams/Carbs: 81
grams

Bursting with flavors and nutritious ingredients, this falafel wrap makes the perfect spring or summer lunch. Two of the main ingredients in this recipe are chickpeas and zucchini. Chickpeas are high in protein which is required for building and repairing tissue in the body. Zucchini is full of beneficial nutrients including fiber, folate and potassium which contribute to a healthy heart.

Ingredients for the Falafel Patties
- 1 can of rinses and drained chickpeas (14 ounces)
- 1 grated zucchini
- 2 minced scallions
- 2 tablespoons of chopped and pitted black olives (optional
- 1 tablespoon of apple cider vinegar or lemon juice
- ½ a teaspoon of ground cumin
- 1 teaspoon of paprika
- 1 /4 teaspoon of sea salt
- 1 teaspoon of olive oil (if frying)

Ingredients for the Wrap

- 1 whole grain pita or wrap
- ¼ cup of classic hummus
- ½ a cup of fresh greens
- 1 baked falafel patty
- ¼ cup of halved cherry tomatoes
- ¼ cup of diced cucumber
- ¼ cup of guacamole or chopped avocado
- 1 cup of cooked quinoa

Directions to Make the Falafel

1. Put the olives (if using), parsley, scallions, zucchini and chickpeas in the food processor and pulse until roughly chopped.
2. In a small bowl, combine the salt, paprika, cumin, lemon juice or apple cider vinegar and tahini and whisk together thoroughly.
3. Pour the mixture into the chickpea mixture and pulse in the food processor.
4. Form the ingredients into 6 patties using your hands.
5. You can either bake the patties or fry them.
6. To bake the patties, line a baking sheet with parchment paper and bake at 350 degrees for 35 minutes.
7. To fry the patties, heat the olive oil in a frying pan and cook on one side for 10 minutes and then on the other side for 5 to 7 minutes.

Directions to Make the Wrap

1. Place the wrap on the plate and spread the hummus down the center.
2. Arrange the greens over the top.
3. Crumble the falafel patty over the top of the greens.
4. Add the quinoa, avocado, cucumber and tomatoes.
5. Fold both ends of the patty and wrap it tightly. You can also press it in a sandwich press if you have one.

GINGER-CASHEW NOODLE SOBA BOWL

Cooking Time: 25 Minutes - Servings: 2 Servings
Calories: 392/Protein: 12 grams/Fat: 28 grams/Carbs: 31
grams

This perfectly healthy dish will fill you up without weighing you down. It makes for the perfect weekend lunch when you don't have much time to spare. Two of the main ingredients are bell peppers and scallions. Bell peppers are packed with vitamins and low in calories. Its vitamin C content is so high that is considered one of the richest dietary sources of this important nutrient.

Ingredients for The Bowls

- 7 ounces of soba noodles
- 1 carrot, julienned and peeled
- 1 bell pepper, thinly sliced and seeded
- 1 cup of snap peas or snow peas, sliced in half and trimmed
- 2 tablespoons of chopped scallions
- 1 cup of chopped lettuce, spinach or kale
- 1 thinly sliced avocado
- 2 tablespoons of chopped cashews

Ingredients for The Dressing

- 1 tablespoon of fresh grated ginger

- 2 tablespoons of cashew butter
- 1 tablespoons of apple cider vinegar
- 2 tablespoons of soy sauce
- 1 teaspoon of toasted sesame oil
- 3 tablespoons of water (optional)

Directions for the Noodles

1. Boil water in a medium sized saucepan according to the instructions on the packet.
2. You can either cook the vegetables or have them raw, if cooking heat some olive oil in a frying pan and sauté the carrots, once they have softened add the bell pepper, the scallions and the peas and then allow them to warm through for one minute before removing them from the heat.

Directions for The Dressing

1. Extract the juice from the grated ginger by squeezing it into a small bowl.
2. Puree all the ingredients together in a food processor and add the water if you want to make it creamier.
3. Lay the bowls with a later of greens, then noodles, drizzle some tamari over the top and add the vegetables.

4. Spoon the dressing over the top, the sliced avocado and then sprinkle the cashews over the top and serve.

RED PEPPER, AVOCADO SUSHI ROLLS

-- You will need a sushi rolling mat for this recipe --

Cooking Time: 1 Hour 15 Minutes - Servings: 4 Servings Calories: 248/Protein: 6 grams/Fat: 7 grams/Carbs: 41 grams

You will never buy sushi from the shop again after you've made this simple but delicious roll. Two of the main ingredients in this recipe are brown rice and alfalfa sprouts. Brown rice contains selenium is a powerful mineral that protects the thyroid against oxidative damage. Alfalfa sprouts are high in vitamin K which helps regulate blood calcium levels.

Ingredients for The Sushi Rice
- 1 cup of brown rice, short grain
- 2 cups of water
- A pinch of salt
- 2 tablespoons of brown rice vinegar

Ingredients for The Sushi Rolls
- 4 nori sheets, standard size of 7 to 8 inches
- 1 thinly sliced avocado
- ¼ thinly sliced red bell pepper
- ¼ cup of alfalfa sprouts

Ingredients to Serve

- Soy or tamari sauce
- 1 tablespoon of pickled ginger
- 1 teaspoon of wasabi

Directions to Make the Sushi Rice

1. Cook the rice according to the directions on the packet and add the salt.
2. Spoon the rice out into a large bowl and leave it to cool down completely.
3. Add just enough vinegar until the rice starts to stick together, sprinkle some salt over the top.

Directions to Make the Sushi Rolls

1. Put a small bowl of water to one side.
2. Arrange the nori sheets rough side up on a rolling mat, the long side should be parallel to you.
3. Wet your hands slightly and place a small handful of rice onto the nori.
4. Spread the rice over the sheet and leave a space of 1 inch along the top edge with no rice.
5. Along the bottom edge, lay a row of avocado slices, then the bell peppers, and then the sprouts.
6. The veggies should fill about one third of the nori sheet.

7. Dry your hands and roll the bottom of the rolling mat over the vegetables. As you roll, press tightly back towards you, and slightly press down on the roll to make sure that its tight.
8. Dip one finger in water and pick up the back end of the rolling mat. Run your finger along the top edge of the nori with no rice.
9. When you have finished rolling, the bare edged seals should be against the outside of the roll.
10. Place the roll back over the mat and help it to seal by gently compressing the roll.
11. Leave the sushi roll to sit for a about 10 minutes so that the rice can soften the nori and then slice into 6 to 8 pieces.
12. Serve with some wasabi, a pickled ginger and a dipping bowl of tamari.

ARTICHOKE AND WHITE BEAN SANDWICH

Cooking Time: 20 Minutes - Servings: 2 Servings
Calories: 110/Protein: 6 grams/Fat: 4 grams/Carbs: 14
grams

This thick juicy sandwich is bursting at the seams with artichoke and creamy smashed white bean. The two main ingredients in this recipe are artichoke and cashew nuts. Artichokes are high in fiber; one medium artichoke contains around 7 grams of fiber which is between 23-28% of the recommended daily intake. Cashew nuts are high in magnesium which supports healthy bones and muscles and protects against high blood pressure.

Ingredients
- 75 grams of raw cashew nuts
- 1 clove of garlic
- 1 teaspoon of fresh rosemary
- ¼ teaspoon of salt
- ¼ teaspoon of black pepper
- The zest of 1 lemon, finely grated
- 6 tablespoons of non-dairy milk
- 1 can of artichoke hearts (150 grams)
- 270 grams of cooked white beans
- ¼ cup of roasted hulled sunflower seeds
- 4 slices of whole wheat bread

Directions

1. Soak the cashew nuts for 15 minutes in boiling water.
2. Add the cashew nuts, milk, lemon zest, salt, pepper, rosemary and garlic to a food processor and blend until all the ingredients are smooth.
3. Pour the beans into a bowl and mash them up with a fork.
4. Add the sunflower seeds and artichoke hearts and continue to mash until combined.
5. Pour the cashew dressing over the top and stir together thoroughly.
6. Arrange the bread on a plate, layer with lettuce, spread the filling over the top and serve.

EGG SALAD SANDWICH

*Cooking Time: 20 Minutes - Servings: 2 Servings
Calories: 248/Protein: 12 grams/Fat: 19 grams/Carbs: 6
grams*

You will never know you are not eating a real egg sandwich! The two main ingredients in this recipe are tofu and romaine lettuce. Tofu is high in protein which is an important building block for blood, skin, cartilage, muscles and bones. Romaine lettuce is high in potassium which helps maintain cardiovascular health.

Ingredients

- 1 block of drained and pat dried medium-firm tofu
- 6 tablespoons of vegan mayonnaise
- 2 tablespoons of nutritional yeast
- 2 tablespoons of yellow mustard
- 2 chopped green onions
- ¾ teaspoons of black salt
- ¼ teaspoon of turmeric
- Salt and pepper
- 8 slices of whole wheat bread
- 4 romaine lettuce leaves

Directions

1. Chop the tofu into small cubes and add it to a large bowl.
2. Add the turmeric, black salt, green onions, yellow mustard, nutritional yeast, mayonnaise and salt and pepper to taste, stir to combine.
3. Arrange the bread on plates, and top with the lettuce, top with the egg salad, and then the other slices of bread and serve.

TOMATO AND CUCUMBER ON TOAST

Cooking Time: 5 Minutes - Servings: 1 Serving
Calories: 177/Protein 3 grams/Fat: 8 grams/Carbs: 3 grams

You won't get more crunchier than cucumber on toast! Combined with the tangy flavor of balsamic vinegar and juicy tomatoes, this five-minute lunch will take you to heaven and back. The two main ingredients in this recipe are cucumber and tomato. Tomatoes are high in the antioxidant lycopene which protect the body against cancer and heart disease. Cucumbers assist in the weight loss process because they are low in calories and have a high-water content.

Ingredients

- 1 teaspoon of balsamic vinegar
- ½ a teaspoon of dried oregano
- ½ a diced cucumber
- ½ a diced tomato
- 2 slices of whole-grain flatbread
- ½ a teaspoon of salt
- ¼ teaspoon of thyme
- ½ a teaspoon of black pepper
- 1 teaspoon of olive oil

Directions

1. In a small bowl, combine the cucumber, tomato, dill, thyme, oregano, olive oil, season with salt and pepper and stir to combine.
2. Arrange the flatbread onto plates and spoon the filling over the top.
3. Fold the flatbread over and serve.

OKRA AND CORN CASSEROLE

*Cooking Time: 55 Minutes - Servings: 6 Servings
Calories: 125/Protein: 4 grams/Fat: 2 grams/Carbs: 17
grams*

This mouth-watering casserole will keep you full until lunchtime. The two main ingredients in this recipe are okra and corn. Okra contains pectin which improves cardiac function by lowering bad cholesterol levels. Corn is high in vitamin B12 which is essential for brain function and nerve tissue health.

Ingredients

- 1 pound of okra
- 1 clove of sliced garlic
- 1 tablespoon of chopped parsley
- 3 tablespoons of olive oil
- 2 large diced tomatoes
- 1 sliced green bell pepper
- 1 can of corn, whole kernel
- 1 small sliced onion

Directions

1. Preheat the oven to 375 degrees F.
2. Slice the okra into small chunks.
3. Heat the olive oil in a medium sized saucepan.

4. Cook the green pepper, okra, onion and garlic for ten minutes, stirring occasionally.
5. Add the tomatoes and the parsley and cook for a further ten minutes.
6. Add the corn and stir to combine.
7. Transfer the ingredients into a baking dish, don't put a lid on it and bake for 30 minutes.
8. Remove from the oven, divide into dishes and serve.

BEAN BOLOGNESE

Cooking Time: 40 Minutes - Servings: 4 Servings
Calories: 442/Protein: 18 grams/Fat: 11 grams/Carbs: 68
grams

Fiber rich beans replace the pork and beef in this tasty meal. The two main ingredients in this recipe are white beans and tomatoes. White beans are a rich source of protein which accelerates the fat burning process. Tomatoes contain beta-carotene which are good for eye health.

Ingredients

- 1 can of white beans (14 ounces) rinsed and drained
- 8 ounces of whole wheat fettuccini
- 1 small chopped onion
- 2 tablespoons of olive oil
- ¼ cup of fresh parsley, chopped and divided
- 1 can of diced tomatoes (14 ounces)
- ½ a cup of balsamic vinegar
- ¼ cup of chopped celery
- ½ a cup of chopped carrots
- 1 bay leaf
- 2 tablespoons of minced garlic
- ½ a teaspoon of salt

Directions

1. Cook the pasta according to the instructions on the packet.
2. Heat the olive oil in a medium sized saucepan and cook the garlic, celery, onion and carrot.
3. Add the salt and the bay leaf and stir for one minute.
4. Add the balsamic vinegar and boil for a further five minutes.
5. Add two tablespoons of parsley, tomatoes and beans, stir to combine and leave the ingredients to simmer for five minutes.
6. Divide the pasta into bowls, spoon the bean bolognase over the top and serve.

CHAPTER 9:
EAT YOUR GREENS - PROTEIN-PACKED SALADS AND DRESSINGS

TUNA SALAD

Cooking Time: 10 Minutes - Servings: 4 Servings
Calories: 298/Protein: 13 grams/Fat: 10 grams/Carbs: 42
grams/Fiber: 13 grams

A crispy, creamy salad that can easily be mistaken for real tuna. The two main ingredients in this recipe are chickpeas and avocados. Chickpeas are a rich source of potassium which lowers blood pressure and protects against loss of muscle mass.

Ingredients

- 1 teaspoon of garlic powder
- ½ a teaspoon of maple syrup
- 1 ½ teaspoons of freshly squeezed lemon juice
- 2 tablespoons of Dijon mustard
- ¼ cup of chopped celery
- ½ a cup of chopped red onion
- 1 pitted and peeled avocado
- A head of romaine lettuce, sliced

Directions

1. Combine the avocado and chickpeas in a large bowl and use a potato masher to smash them down.

2. Add the garlic powder, maple syrup, lemon juice, mustard, celery and onion and stir to combine.

3. Divide the lettuce onto plates, spoon the tuna salad over the top and serve.

SOUTHWEST SPINACH SALAD

Cooking Time: 10 Minutes - Servings: 2 Servings
Calories: 197/Protein: 11 grams/Fat: 4 grams/Carbs: 34
grams/Fiber: 10 grams

This satisfying salad can be eaten as main course or as a tasty side dish. The two main ingredients in this recipe are spinach and brown rice.

Ingredients

- ½ a tablespoon of flaxseeds
- ½ a cup of corn
- ½ a cup of cooked brown rice
- ½ a cup of cooked black beans
- 8 ounces of fresh spinach
- ¼ teaspoon of red pepper flakes
- ½ a teaspoon of smoked paprika
- ½ a teaspoon of BBQ sauce
- ½ a teaspoon of balsamic vinegar

Directions

1. Combine the BBQ sauce, red pepper flakes, paprika and vinegar in a large bowl and whisk to combine.
2. Add the corn, rice, black beans and spinach and toss to coat.
3. Divide onto plates, top with flaxseed and serve.

KALE AND LEMON SALAD

Cooking Time: 10 Minutes - Servings: 4 Servings
Calories: 51/Protein: 3 grams/Fat: 0 grams/Carbs: 11
grams/Fiber: 1 gram

This citrus-filled crispy salad is great for those warm summer BBQ months. The main ingredients in this recipe are kale and lemon.

Ingredients

- 5 cups of chopped kale
- 1 teaspoon of minced garlic
- ½ a tablespoon of maple syrup
- 2 tablespoons of lemon juice, freshly squeezed

Directions

1. Combine the garlic, maple syrup and lemon juice in a large bowl and whisk to combine.
2. Add the kale and massage the dressing into it for two minutes before serving.

MANGO JICAMA BASIL SALAD

*Cooking Time: 1 Hour 15 Minutes - Servings: 6 Servings
Calories: 76/Protein: 1 grams/Fat: 2 grams/Carbs: 14
grams*

If you've never had the pleasure of tasting jicama, you are in for a treat! This recipe uses basil and mango for a highly favorable and tropical meal. The two main ingredients are jicama and mango. Jicama is packed with fiber which lowers cholesterol and prevents constipation. Mangoes contain enzymes that assist in the breakdown of fiber and protein.

Ingredients

- 1 jicama, grated and peeled
- 1 peeled and sliced mango
- ¼ cup of non-dairy milk
- 2 tablespoons of chopped, fresh basil
- 1 large chopped scallion
- ¼ teaspoon of sea salt
- 1 ½ tablespoons of tahini (optional)
- Fresh greens (to serve)
- Chopped cashews (to serve, optional)
- Cheesy sprinkle (to serve, optional)

Directions

1. Place the jicama into a large bowl.
2. Add the milk and mango to a food processor and blend until smooth.
3. Add the scallions, basil, tahini and salt and continue to blend.
4. Add the dressing to the jicama, stir to combine, put a lid on the bowl and refrigerate for an hour.
5. Arrange the greens on a plate, add the jicama and sprinkle the cheesy sprinkle and cashews over the top and serve.

AVOCADO AND ROASTED BEET SALAD

Cooking Time: 40 Minutes - Servings: 2 Servings
Calories: 167/Protein: 4 grams/Fat: 13 grams/Carbs: 15
grams

We all love beetroot and avocado on their own, but the two combined is absolutely divine! The two main ingredients in this recipe are beets and avocados. Beets contain dietary nitrates which enhance athletic performance. Avocados are a great source of vitamin E which prevents inflammation in the body and supports eye health.

Ingredients

- 2 beets, thinly sliced and peeled
- 1 teaspoon of olive oil
- A pinch of sea salt
- 1 avocado
- 2 cups of mixed greens
- 4 tablespoons of creamy Balsamic Dressing
- 2 tablespoons of chopped almonds

Directions

1. Prepare the oven by preheating it to 450 degrees F.
2. In a large bowl, combine the oil, beets and salt, massage with your hands.

3. Arrange the beets in a single layer on a baking dish and bake them for 30 minutes.

4. Slice the avocado in half and remove the seed.

5. Scoop out the avocado flesh in one piece and slice it into crescents.

6. Once the beets are cooked, remove them from the oven and arrange the slices onto plates.

7. Top the beets with a slice of avocado, a handful of salad and drizzle the dressing over the top, coat with some chopped almonds and serve.

KALE SALAD WITH CREAMY AVOCADO

Cooking Time: 30 Minutes - Servings: 4 Servings
Calories: 225/Protein: 7 grams/Fat: 7 grams/Carbs: 37
grams

You will never taste a better kale salad! The lemon juice and avocado and scallions add a nice touch. The main two main ingredients are kale and millet. Kale is loaded with powerful antioxidants such as kaempferol and quercetin which reduce inflammation, lower blood pressure and protect the heart. Millet is rich in phosphorus which protect the kidneys by assisting in the waste filtering process.

Ingredients for the Dressing
- 1 peeled and pitted avocado
- 1 tablespoon of fresh lemon juice
- 1 tablespoon of fresh dill
- 1 small clove of garlic, pressed
- 1 chopped scallion
- A pinch of sea salt
- ¼ cup of water

Ingredients for the Salad
- 8 large leaves of kale
- ½ a cup of chopped green beans
- 1 cup of halved cherry tomatoes

- 1 chopped, bell pepper
- 2 chopped scallions
- 2 cups of cooked millet
- Hummus (optional)

Directions to Make the Dressing

1. Transfer all the ingredients into a food processor, and blend until smooth.
2. You can add more salt if you need to.

Directions to Make the Salad

1. Remove the stems from the kale and chop the leaves. Add a pinch of salt and massage with your fingers to soften the kale.
2. In a large bowl combine the millet, scallions, bell pepper, cherry tomatoes, green beans, kale and the dressing, toss to combine all ingredients.
3. Arrange the salad onto plates, if using hummus, place a spoonful on the side of each plate.

AUBERGINE MOROCCAN SALAD

Cooking Time: 45 Minutes - Servings: 2 Servings
Calories: 97/Protein: 4 grams/Fat: 4 grams/Carbs: 16
grams

This velvety aubergine salad provides a gentle boost of Moroccan flavor. The two main ingredients in this recipe are aubergine and eggplant. Aubergines contain an antioxidant called nasunin which protects the fats in the brain. Eggplant contains magnesium which helps transport blood sugar into the muscles which boosts exercise performance.

Ingredients

- 1 teaspoon of olive oil
- 1 diced egg plant
- ½ a teaspoon of ground cumin
- ½ a teaspoon of ground ginger
- ¼ teaspoon of turmeric
- ¼ teaspoon of ground nutmeg
- A pinch of sea salt
- The juice and zest of half a lemon
- Half a lemon sliced into wedges
- 2 tablespoons of capers
- 1 tablespoon of green olives chopped
- 1 clove of garlic, pressed

- A handful of finely chopped fresh mint
- 2 cups of chopped spinach

Directions

1. In a large frying pan, heat the oil over a medium temperature.
2. Sauté the eggplant for 5 minutes and then add the nutmeg, turmeric, ginger, cumin and salt, and stir to combine. Continue to cook for about 10 minutes until the eggplant becomes extremely soft.
3. Add the mint, garlic, olives, capers, lemon juice and zest.
4. Arrange a handful of spinach onto each plate and top with the eggplant mixture.
5. Squeeze a wedge of lemon over the top and serve.

POTATO AND DILL SALAD

Cooking Time: 35 Minutes - Servings: 4 Servings
Calories: 246/Protein: 8 grams/Fat: 1 grams/Carbs: 55
grams

Everyone loves potato salad, this recipe is creamy, rich and loaded with fresh dill. The two main ingredients in this meal are potatoes and zucchini. Potatoes contain niacin which helps to boost brain function and lowers bad cholesterol levels.

Ingredients

- 6 medium potatoes sliced into cubes
- 1 zucchini sliced into cubes
- ¼ cup of fresh dill, chopped
- 2 teaspoons of Dijon mustard
- 1/8 teaspoon of sea salt
- Ground black pepper
- 1 teaspoon of nutritional yeast (optional)
- Milk – the non-dairy kind (optional)
- 3 chopped stalks of celery
- 1 bell pepper chopped and seeded
- 1 tablespoon of scallions, chopped

Directions

1. Boil a large pot of water, add the potatoes and boil for 10 minutes.

2. Add the zucchini and boil for a further 10 minutes.

3. Take the saucepan off the fire, drain the water, but save one cup of the water.

4. Transfer the potatoes and zucchini in a bowl and set to one side to cool down.

5. Put ½ a cup of the potatoes and zucchini into a food processor, add the water from step 3, nutritional yeast (if using), salt, pepper, mustard, dill, non-dairy milk (if using) and blend until smooth.

6. Add the chives, bell pepper and celery to the rest of the zucchini and potatoes, pour the dressing over the top, arrange onto plates and serve.

WHITE BEAN TUSCAN SALAD

Cooking Time: 40 Minutes - Servings: 2 Servings
Calories: 360/Protein: 18 grams/Fat: 8 grams/Carbs: 68
grams

This simple summer side dish is a great choice on for those days when you don't want to cook a full meal. The two main ingredients are cannellini beans and mushrooms. Cannellini beans are an excellent source of protein helps to build muscle mass and boost strength. Mushrooms contain vitamin D which is required to help the body absorb calcium.

Ingredients for Then Dressing
- 1 tablespoon of olive oil
- 2 tablespoons of balsamic vinegar
- 1 tablespoon of scallions, minced
- 1 clove of minced garlic
- 1 tablespoon of chopped, fresh rosemary
- 1 tablespoon of chopped, fresh oregano
- A pinch of salt

Ingredients for The Salad
- 1 can of cannellini beans, rinsed and drained
- 6 thinly sliced mushrooms
- 1 diced zucchini
- 2 diced carrots
- 2 tablespoons of chopped, fresh basil

Directions

1. To make the dressing, add all the ingredients into a food processor and blend until smooth.
2. Arrange the salad in a plastic container, pour the dressing over the top, toss to combine, cover and refrigerate for 30 minutes before serving.

EDAMAME AND BLACK RICE SALAD

Cooking Time: 40 Minutes - Servings: 4 Servings
Calories: 445/Protein: 15 grams/Fat: 11 grams/Carbs: 75
grams

This unique and tasty salad recipe will have you and your guests going back for seconds. The two main ingredients in this recipe are black rice and edamame beans. Black rice contains phytonutrients which cleanse the body of toxins. Edamame beans are a whole protein source which provide the body with all the essential amino acids it needs.

Ingredients for The Salad

- 1 cup of black rice
- 2 cups of water
- A pinch of sea salt
- 1 large sweet potato
- 1 teaspoon of olive oil
- 1 cup of edamame beans
- 1 chopped and seeded bell pepper
- ½ a head of chopped broccoli
- 4 chopped scallions
- Chopped fresh cilantro
- Sesame seeds

Ingredients for The Dressing

- The juice of ½ an orange
- 1 tablespoon of soy sauce
- 1 tablespoon of apple cider vinegar
- 2 teaspoons of maple syrup
- 2 teaspoons of sesame oil

Directions

1. Prepare the oven by preheating it to 400 degrees F.
2. Cook the rice according to the instructions on the packet. Once the rice is cooked, remove it from the stove, drain and rinse the rice and set it to one side to cool down.
3. Peel the sweet potato, dice it and toss olive oil over the top.
4. Arrange the sweet potato over a baking dish and bake for 20 minutes. Once cooked, remove them from the oven and leave them to cool down.
5. Transfer all the ingredients for the dressing into a jar and shake to combine.
6. In a large bowl, add the scallions, broccoli, bell pepper, edamame, sweet potato and rice and toss to combine.
7. Arrange onto plates, drizzle the dressing over the top, and garnish with sesame seeds and fresh cilantro.

SWEET DILL DRESSING

Cooking Time: 5 Minutes - Servings: 1 cup
Calories: /Protein: grams/Fat: grams/Carbs: grams

This tangy dressing makes a tasty topping for any salad. The two main ingredients in this recipe are apple cider vinegar and dill. Apple cider vinegar kills several harmful bacteria and lowers cholesterol. Dill is high in vitamin A which helps support a healthy immune system.

Ingredients

- 3 tablespoons of water
- ¼ teaspoon of garlic powder
- 1 teaspoon of dried dill
- 1 tablespoon of apple cider vinegar
- 1 tablespoon of agave nectar
- 3 tablespoons of veganaise
- ¼ cup of nutritional yeast

Directions

1. Combine all the ingredients in a food processor and blend until smooth.

CHERRY TOMATO DRESSING

Cooking Time: 5 Minutes - Servings: 1 Cup
Calories: 54 /Protein: 0.3 grams/Fat: 1.2 grams/Carbs: 3 grams

If this is your first batch of cherry tomato dressing, I can guarantee that it won't be your last. The two main ingredients in this recipe are cherry tomatoes and balsamic vinegar. Tomatoes contain potassium which helps to build muscle strength and helps keep the brain healthy. Balsamic vinegar contains acetic acid which contain probiotics which promote good gut health.

Ingredients

- ¼ teaspoon of black pepper
- ¼ teaspoon of salt
- ¼ teaspoon of garlic powder
- ½ teaspoon of onion powder
- ½ a teaspoon of paprika
- 1 tablespoon of agave nectar
- ¼ cup of olive oil
- ¼ cup of balsamic vinegar
- Cherry tomatoes

Directions

1. Combine all the ingredients in a food processor and blend until smooth.

GREEK DRESSING

Cooking Time: 5 Minutes - Servings: 1 Cup
Calories: 35 /Protein: 4 grams/Fat: 0.2 grams/Carbs: 4.5
grams

A dressing fit enough for a king! The two main ingredients in this recipe are oregano and lemon. Oregano helps regulate blood sugar and fight bacteria. Lemons are a good source of vitamin C which help to promote heart health.

Ingredients

- ¼ teaspoon of black pepper
- ¼ teaspoon of salt
- ¼ teaspoon of garlic powder
- ½ teaspoon of dried oregano
- 1 tablespoon of Dijon mustard
- ¼ cup of lemon juice
- ¼ cup of olive oil

Directions

1. Combine all the ingredients in a food processor and blend until smooth.

MUSTARD MAPLE DRESSING

Cooking Time: 5 Minutes - Servings: 1 Cup
Calories: 24 /Protein: 0.1 grams/Fat: 4 grams/Carbs: 6
grams

A simple yet delicious dressing bursting with flavors. The two main ingredients in this recipe are mustard and maple syrup. Mustard is a rich source of calcium which is required to build and maintain strong bones.

Ingredients

- ¼ teaspoon of garlic powder
- 1 tablespoon of lemon juice
- 2 tablespoons of Dijon mustard
- 2 tablespoons of maple syrup
- ¼ cup of olive oil

Directions

1. Combine all the ingredients into a food processor and blend until smooth.

CHAPTER 10:
THE PRE AND POST WORKOUT
SNACKS YOU NEED TO BE EATING

PRE-WORKOUT

LOADED BAKED POTATOES

*Cooking Time: 1 Hour 30 Minutes - Servings: 4 Servings
Calories: 75 /Protein: 4.2 grams/Fat: 6 grams/Carbs: 67
grams/Fiber: 4.7 grams*

This mouth-watering loaded jacket potato makes the perfect pre-workout meal! The two main ingredients for this recipe are potatoes and kidney beans. Potatoes contain calcium which protect the body against high blood pressure and diabetes. Kidney beans are high in fiber which promotes colon health and assists in the weight loss process.

Ingredients

1. 1 small handful of chopped chives
2. 1 batch of vegan nacho cheese
3. ½ a cup of vegan BBQ sauce
4. 1 can of kidney beans
5. 1 tablespoon of olive oil
6. 4 russet potatoes

Directions

1. Prepare the oven by heating it to 350 degrees F.
2. Use a fork to poke holes in the potatoes and rub them with olive oi.
3. Put the potatoes in the center of the rack and bake for 1 hour 30 minutes.
4. The jacket potatoes are ready when you can easily pierce them all the way through with a knife.
5. Prepare the cheese according to the instructions on the packet.
6. Combine the kidney beans and the BBQ sauce in a saucepan and let the mixture cook for approximately 5 minutes.
7. Remove the jacket potatoes from the oven, slice them down the middle and top with the kidney beans, pour the cheese over the top, garnish with the chives and serve.

OVERNIGHT OATS

Cooking Time: 8 Hours - Servings: 1 Servings
Calories: 43 /Protein: 7.8 grams/Fat: 3.2 grams/Carbs: 2.1
grams/Fiber: 5.6 grams

This delicious pre workout meal works just as well as a breakfast. The two main ingredients in this recipe are bananas and oats. Bananas protect the body against kidney disorders, and it helps to build muscle strength. Oats contain a powerful soluble fiber called beta glucan which regulates cholesterol levels and boosts heart health.

Ingredients

- A handful of blueberries
- Maple syrup
- ¼ teaspoon of cinnamon
- ¼ cup of chopped strawberries
- ½ a diced banana
- ½ a cup of plant milk
- ½ a cup of oats

Directions

1. Combine the milk, maple syrup, cinnamon and oats in a bowl and stir to combine. Leave it in the fridge overnight.
2. The next morning add the bananas, strawberries and blueberries and serve.

BANANA ICE-CREAM

Cooking Time: 20 Minutes - Servings: 2 Servings Calories: 21/Protein: 3.1 grams/Fat: 8 grams/Carbs: 12.1 grams/Fiber: 3 grams

The wonderful thing about this ice-cream is that it's delicious enough to eat without a topping. The main ingredients in this recipe are bananas and peanuts. Bananas contain manganese which helps to improve bone health. Peanuts contain phosphorous which helps the body store and use energy.

Ingredients

- 4 ripe bananas
- ½ a cup of shelled peanuts
- 2 tablespoons of maple syrup
- Sea salt

Directions

1. Prepare the oven by heating it to 350 degrees F.
2. Place parchment paper over a baking tray.
3. Roughly chop the peanuts and spread them out onto the baking tray.
4. Drizzle the maple syrup over the top of the peanuts and season with some sea salt.
5. Bake the peanuts for 10 minutes.

6. Remove the peanuts from the oven and allow them to cool down.

7. Blend the frozen bananas in a food processor until smooth.

8. Spoon the banana ice-cream into bowls, top with the roasted peanuts and serve.

RAW CHOCOLATE PUDDING WITH CARDAMOM BLUEBERRY SAUCE

Cooking Time: 20 Minutes - Servings: 2
Calories: 67 /Protein: 4.2 grams/Fat: 3 grams/Carbs: 5.4 grams

If you are a fan of delicious health-giving foods, this one is for you! A delicious assortment of bananas, chocolate and peanut butter, it can't get any yummier! The two main ingredients in this recipe are avocado and banana. Avocados are a good source of riboflavin which is required to assist the body in breaking down proteins and carbohydrates. Bananas are high in the trace mineral manganese which is required for the normal functioning of the nervous system and the brain.

Ingredients for The Chocolate Pudding
- 2 avocados, ripe
- 1 large banana, ripe
- ½ a cup of cacao powder
- ½ a cup of natural peanut butter
- 4 dates, pitted
- Non-dairy milk (if necessary)

Ingredients for The Cardamom Blueberry Sauce
- 1 cup of blueberries, fresh or frozen

- 2 dates, pitted
- 1 tablespoon of maple syrup
- ½ a teaspoon of cinnamon
- The zest of 1 lemon
- A pinch of cardamom

Directions for The Chocolate Pudding

1. Transfer all ingredients into a food processor and blend until smooth and creamy.
2. You can add some non-dairy milk to thin it out if you need to.
3. Divide into little serving classes, place plastic wrap over the top and leave it to chill in the fridge overnight.
4. Remove from the fridge the next day, top with the sauce and serve.

Directions for The Cardamom Blueberry Sauce

1. Transfer all the ingredients into a food processor and blend until smooth.

RAW CHOCOLATE CHIP DOUGH BITE COOKIES

Cooking Time: 20 Minutes - Servings: 2
Calories: 41/Protein: 6.7 grams/Fat: 2.4 grams/Carbs: 3.2 grams

Not only is this a comfort snack, it's also totally healthy. The two main ingredients in this recipe are cashews and dark chocolate. Cashews support heart health by lowering bad cholesterol. Dark chocolate is a powerful source of antioxidants which protect the body against free radical damage.

Ingredients

- 1 cup of cashews, raw
- ½ a cup of whole oat
- 8 pitted dates
- ½ a teaspoon of Himalayan salt
- ¼ teaspoon of raw vanilla powder
- 2 tablespoons of dark chocolate sliced into small pieces

Directions

1. Put the oats and cashews into a food processor and blend until combined but still chunky.
2. Add the pitted dates and pulse for a few seconds.

3. Add the vanilla powder and the Himalayan salt and pulse for a further 30 seconds.
4. Add the chocolate and pulse until combined.
5. Shape the dough into your desired shape, (bars, squares, circles etc.), store them in a separate freezer bags and freeze.
6. Remove the bars from the fridge when you are ready to eat them.

ROASTED CHICKPEAS

Cooking Time: 30 Minutes - Servings:
Calories: 21 /Protein: 3.4 grams/Fat: 5 grams/Carbs: 3
grams

This tasty crunchy snack makes a delightful pre workout treat. The two main ingredients are chickpeas and olive oil. Chickpeas are an excellent source of plant-based proteins which assist in the weight loss process and help to prevent diabetes.

Ingredients

- 2 cans of chickpeas
- 2 tablespoons of olive oil
- Any seasoning you wish (see suggestions below)

Directions

1. Prepare the oven by preheating it to 375 degrees F.
2. Drain and rinse the beans and then dry them out on a towel until any extra moisture has been absorbed.
3. Line a baking sheet with parchment paper and arrange the chickpeas onto the tray.

4. Roast the chickpeas for 45-60 minutes (make sure they are crunchy before removing them from the oven).

5. As soon as the chickpeas are cooked, toss them with olive oil and the seasoning you want to use.

6. They are best served hot.

--Seasoning Suggestions—

Spice Smokey Blend

- ½ a teaspoon of sea salt
- ¼ teaspoon of black pepper
- ½ a teaspoon of cumin
- ½ a teaspoon of garlic powder
- ½ a teaspoon of smoked paprika
- ½ a teaspoon of ancho chili powder
- A pinch of cayenne pepper

Parmesan Garlic

- ¼cup of parmesan cheese, grated
- 1 teaspoon of garlic powder
- ¼ teaspoon of black pepper
- ½ a teaspoon of salt

Cinnamon Honey

- 2 tablespoons of honey
- ¼ teaspoon of sea salt
- A pinch of nutmeg

- 1 teaspoon of cinnamon
- After coating the chickpeas in the cinnamon honey, put them back in the oven for 15 minutes to caramelize

Soy Sesame
- 1 tablespoon of sesame seeds
- ½ a teaspoon of sea salt
- 1 teaspoon of garlic powder
- 1 teaspoon of sesame oil

RUSH MATCHA SMOOTHIE

*Cooking Time: 10 Minutes - Servings:
Calories: 31 /Protein: 3.3 grams/Fat: 2 grams/Carbs: 5.6
grams*

Tastes like a creamy milkshake but it's filled with yummy goodness. The two main ingredients in this recipe are matcha powder and banana. Matcha is packed with antioxidants, speeds up the metabolism and burns calories. Bananas provide powerful energy boosting components.

Ingredients

- 1 cup of non-dairy milk of your choice
- 1 banana, frozen
- 1 teaspoon of matcha powder, organic
- 2 pitted medjool dates
- 1 tablespoon of almond butter
- 1 tablespoon of vegan protein powder
- A pinch of Celtic sea salt

Directions

1. Transfer all the ingredients into a food processor and blend until smooth. Add milk according to your preference for consistency.

RAW AND SIMPLE GRANOLA

Cooking Time: 5 Minutes - Servings: 3 cups
Calories: 139 /Protein: 4.4 grams/Fat: 9.7 grams/Carbs:
10.9 grams

This is the only raw plant-based granola recipe you will ever needs! The two main ingredients in this recipe are figs and coconut. Figs are a rich source of copper which is required for to maintain the immune system. Coconuts contain selenium which help prevent against mental decline.

Ingredients

- 1 teaspoon of cinnamon
- 6 figs, dried and chopped
- ¼ cup of goji berries
- ¼ cup of raisins
- ¼ cup of raw cashews
- ¼ cup of pumpkin seeds
- ¼ cup of sunflower seeds
- ¼ cup of chia seeds
- ¼ cup of flaxseeds
- 1 cup of coconut, shredded
- 1/3 cup of cacao butter
- 1/3 cup of agave syrup

Directions

1. Soak the cashews, pumpkin seeds and sunflower seeds in a jar full of room temperature water overnight.
2. Soak the goji berries and the raisins in a separate bowl and soak them in water for 15 minutes.
3. Drain and rinse the seeds in a fine mesh metal strainer.
4. Do the same for the goji berries and the raisins.
5. Combine the figs, goji berries, raisins, cashews, pumpkin seeds, sunflower seeds, chia seeds, flax seeds, coconut, cinnamon and salt in a large bowl and toss to combine.
6. Chop up the cacao butter into small chunks and heat it in a saucepan until it melts. Remove the saucepan from the stove an allow it to cool down completely.
7. Add the agave syrup and whisk to combine.
8. Pour the sauce on top of the dry ingredients and use a spatula to mix the ingredients together.
9. Place a lid over the bowl and refrigerate for 1-2 hours.
10. Pour the granola into a glass jar and keep it in the fridge for no longer than 2 weeks.

TABBOULEH SALAD

*Cooking Time: 20 Minutes - Servings: 2 Servings
Calories: 105/Protein: 2.7 grams/Fat: 3.8 grams/Carbs:
16.7 grams*

A healthy and fresh salad made with herbs and bulgur wheat. The two main ingredients in this recipe are bulgur wheat and parsley. Bulgur wheat contains iron which is required to regulate body temperature. Parsley is made up of antibacterial properties which help the body fight disease.

Ingredients

- 2 bunches of finely chopped fresh Italian parsley
- 4 finely chopped large tomatoes
- The juice of 3 lemons
- 5 tablespoons of olive oil
- 1 cup of boiled water
- 5 tablespoons of olive oil
- 1 cup of bulgur
- 1/8 teaspoon of ground black pepper
- 1/8 teaspoon of salt

Directions

- In a small bowl, combine the bulgur and the cup of boiled water and stir to combine. Put a tea towel over the bowel and leave it to cook. Once cooked, put remove the tea towel, put it to one side and leave the bulgur to cool down.

- Combine the tomatoes and the parsley in a large salad bowl.
- Pour the lemon juice over the salad mixture.
- Add the black pepper, salt and olive oil and toss to combine.
- Pour the cooled bulgur mix over the top, stir to combine and serve.

JAM AND PEANUT BUTTER STUFFED DATES

Cooking Time: 10 Minutes - Servings: 12 servings
Calories: 114 /Protein: 2 grams/Fat: 3 grams/Carbs: 23
grams

There is nothing better than creamy peanut butter layered with mouthwatering jam and chocolate, all inside sweet and juicy dates! The two main ingredients inside this recipe are dates and dark chocolate. Dates are a rich source of antioxidants and help to reduce blood pressure. Dark chocolate is helps to improve blood flow to the organs in the body.

Ingredients for the Dates
- 12 medjdool dates
- ¼ cup of peanut butter, all natural
- ¼ cup of raspberry chia jam
- 2 tablespoons of dark chocolate, sliced into chunks

Ingredients for The Raspberry Jam
- 1 cup of Fresh or frozen raspberries
- 1 teaspoon of Chia seeds
- A pinch of sea salt
- 2 tablespoons of maple syrup

Directions for The Raspberry Jam

1. Transfer the raspberries into a saucepan and cook them on medium to high heat for 5 minutes until they get soft.
2. Add the maple syrup, chia seeds and salt and stir to combine.
3. Allow the jam to simmer for 2-3 minutes and then remove it from the heat.
4. Leave it to set and thicken for 10 minutes before using.
5. You can store the jam in the fridge for up to 5 days.

Directions for The Dates

1. Cut the dates down the middle in a vertical direction and remove the pits.
2. Fill each date with 1 teaspoon of raspberry jam and one teaspoon of peanut butter.
3. Sprinkle the dark chocolate over the top and serve.

POST-WORKOUT

HONEY TOFU AND GINGER STIR-FRY

Cooking Time: 25 Minutes - Servings: 6 Servings
Calories: 375/Protein: 12 grams/Fat: 14 grams/Carbs: 52.4
grams/Fiber: 4 grams

The perfect treat after a long workout! The two main ingredients in this recipe are brown rice and tofu. Brown rice is packed with fiber which supports colon health. Tofu is a good source of calcium which helps to maintain muscle health.

Ingredients for the Stir Fry

- 3 minced green onions
- 2 cups of shredded carrots
- 2 cups of chopped asparagus
- 14 ounces of extra firm tofu
- 2 tablespoons of canola oil
- 1 ½ cups of brown rice

Ingredients for the Ginger Garlic Stir Fry Sauce

- ¼ cup of canola oil
- ¼ cup of rice wine vinegar
- ¼ cup of water

- ½ a cup of low sodium soy sauce
- 2 tablespoons of honey
- 2 tablespoons of fresh ginger
- 3 cloves of garlic

Directions For the Sauce

1. Combine all the ingredients in a food processor, blend until smooth and set it to one side.

Directions for the Stir Fry

1. Cook the brown rice according to the instructions on the packet and set it to one side.
2. Cut the tofu up and pat dry with a paper towel to get rid of any excess water and then slice into small cubes.
3. In a large frying pan, heat the oil over medium temperature and add the tofu.
4. Add ¼ cup of the stir fry sauce and put a lid on the frying pan and let the tofu fry until it turns golden brown in color.
5. Line a plate with a kitchen towel and transfer the tofu onto the plate.
6. Put the frying pan back on the cooker and add ¼ cup of stir fry sauce and the asparagus. Once it is tender crisp and bright green add the carrots and toss to combine.

7. Spoon the rice out onto plates and top with
    the tofu mix, vegetables, garnish with the
    green onions and serve.

152

LENTIL SPICED BURGER

Cooking Time: 30 Minutes - Servings: 10 Servings Calories: 245/Protein: 30 grams/Fat: 1 gram/Carbs: 30 grams/Fiber: 8 grams

A juicy burger full of rich spicy goodness. The main ingredients in this recipe are lentils and walnuts. Lentils make a low-calorie meat replacement because of their high protein content. Walnuts are rich in antioxidants and help to support the weight loss process.

Ingredients

- Olive oil
- 10 whole grain buns
- 1 teaspoon of fine sea salt
- 1 tablespoon of chopped fresh oregano
- 1 tablespoon of chopped fresh thyme
- 2 tablespoons of vegan Worcestershire sauce
- 2 tablespoons of tomato paste
- 2 flax eggs
- 1 cup of whole grain breadcrumbs
- ½ a cup of chickpea flour
- ½ a cup of sunflower seeds
- ½ a cup of walnuts
- 3 cloves of minced garlic

- 1 cup of finely chopped onions
- 2 ½ cups of cooked green lentils
- 10 pieces of romaine lettuce
- 3 fresh tomatoes, sliced

Directions

1. Combine the sunflower seeds, walnuts, garlic, carrots and onions in a food processor and blend to combine. Transfer the mixture into a large bowl.
2. Blend half of the lentils until they are slightly mashed and add them to the bowl, add the remaining lentils to the bowl and stir to combine the ingredients.
3. Add the herbs, breadcrumbs and the salt.
4. In a separate bowl, combine the tomato paste, flax egg and Worcestershire sauce and whisk to combine.
5. Pour the tomato mixture into the lentil mixture and stir to combine.
6. Add the flour a bit at a time and keep stirring. Once everything is combined, put the mixture in the fridge for 30 minutes to dry it out.
7. Remove the mixture from the fridge and form the patties using your hands.
8. Heat the olive oil in a frying pan over medium heat and start frying the burgers, if you are

not going to use them all, you can leave the mixture in the fridge for up to five days.

9. Toast the buns in a toaster and arrange them on plates. Place the lentil burgers on top, layer with lettuce leaves, tomatoes and vegan mayonnaise and serve.

FLAXSEED YOGURT

Cooking Time: 5 Minutes - Servings: 4 Servings
Calories: 220 /Protein: 10 grams/Fat: 16.9 grams/Carbs:
9.2 grams

A healthy, yet delicious yogurt alternative! The main ingredients in this recipe are hemp seeds and flax seeds. Hemp seeds are rich in essential fatty acids which play a role in heart health. Flax seeds are a rich source of lignans which help reduce the risk of cancer.

Ingredients

- 2 cups of water
- ½ a cup of hemp seeds
- ½ a cup of flax seeds
- 1 cup of almond milk
- 2 teaspoons of psyllium husk
- ¼ cup of lemon juice
- ¼ teaspoon of stevia

Directions

- Put the flaxseeds in a bowl of water, cover and leave them to soak for 10 minutes. Once soaked, drain the water and put them to one side.

- Add a cup of boiling water to a food processor, add the flax seeds and blend for approximately 4 minutes.
- Add a cup of water, the psyllium husk and the almond milk to the food processor and blend for a further 30 seconds.
- Add the stevia and lemon juice and blend for another couple of seconds.
- Transfer the flaxseed yogurt into a sealable container and store in the fridge.
- Eat once chilled.
- You can store the flaxseed yogurt in an airtight container for 3-4 days and or in an airtight container for 60 days in a freezer.

MEXIKALE CHIPS

Cooking Time: 10 Minutes - Servings: 2
Calories: 313 /Protein: 12 grams/Fiber: 7grams/Fat: 14.6
grams/Carbs: 33.4grams

You will never buy another bag of chips again with these Mexican style Kale chips. The two main ingredients in this recipe are kale and nutritional yeast. Kale is an excellent source of vitamin K which is responsible for bone metabolism. Nutritional yeast is high in vitamin B12 which reduces the risk of macular degeneration.

Ingredients

- 8 cups of chopped large kale leaves
- 2 tablespoons of avocado oil
- 2 tablespoons of nutritional yeast
- 1 teaspoon of garlic powder
- 1 teaspoon of ground cumin
- ½ a teaspoon of chili powder
- 1 teaspoon of dried oregano
- Salt and pepper

Directions

1. Prepare the oven by heating it to 350 degrees F.
2. Place parchment paper over a baking tray and put it to one side.

3. Use a paper towel to absorb all the water from the kale leaves.
4. Put the kale leaves into a large bowl, add the seasonings, yeast and avocado oil and toss to combine.
5. Spread the kale onto the baking tray and bake for 10 minutes.
6. If they are not crispy enough, keep checking every 1 minute until they are to your liking.
7. Remove the tray from the oven and set it to one side to cool down before serving.

CHOCOLATE AND HAZELNUT BARS

Cooking Time: 15 minutes - Serves: 4 Servings
Calories: 296 /Protein: 20.6 grams/Fiber: 3 grams/Fat: 14.2
grams/Carbs: 21.3 grams

It will be impossible for you to only eat one of these yummy bars. The two main ingredients in this recipe are hazelnuts and cashew butter. Hazelnuts contain oleic acid which plays a role in maintaining mental health. Cashew butter contains amino acids which are responsible for enhancing muscle growth.

Ingredients

- 1 cup of chocolate protein powder (vegan)
- ¼ cup of chopped hazelnuts
- ¼ cup of cocoa powder, unsweetened
- 1/3 cup of almond milk
- ¼ cup of cashew butter
- 3 tablespoons of brown rice syrup
- Crushed almonds or hazelnuts for garnishing (optional)

Directions

1. Combine the hazelnuts and protein powder in a large bowl and whisk to combine.
2. Add the brown rice syrup, cashew butter, and almond milk and continue to whisk until all

the ingredients are mixed together thoroughly until they form into a dough.

3. Line a baking tray with parchment paper and place the dough in the center of the tray.

4. Use a rolling pin to roll the dough out until it becomes a ½ an inch-thick square.

5. Put the baking tray in the freezer for one hour and a half.

6. Once frozen, slice the square into 8 equal bars, garnish with almonds and hazelnuts if using.

7. You can store the bars in the fridge for one day.

VANILLA CRANBERRY PROTEIN BARS

Cooking Time: 15 Minutes - Serves: 4 Servings
Calories: 243 /Protein: 16.1 grams/Fiber: 3.1 grams/Fat:
9.6 grams/Carbs: 22.9 grams

The combination of vanilla and cranberry make for an irresistible treat. The two main ingredients in this recipe are oats and cranberries. Oats are a rich source of antioxidants that protect the body against free radical damage. Cranberries contain 25% of your daily requirement for vitamin C.

Ingredients

- 1 cup of old-fashioned oats
- 2 cups of vanilla protein powder (vegan)
- ½ a cup of shredded coconut
- ½ a cup of cashew butter
- ½ a cup of dried cranberries
- ¼ cup of maple syrup
- ¼ cup of chia seeds
- 1 tablespoon of almond milk
- 1 tablespoon of pure vanilla extract

Directions

1. Lay parchment paper on a baking dish and put it to one side.

2. Add the shredded coconut, protein powder and oats to a food processor and blend until the ingredients turn into a fine powder.

3. Pour the powdered mixture into a large mixing bowl and add the rest of the ingredients.

4. Whisk the ingredients together until it turns into a dough.

5. Place the dough in the middle of the baking dish and flatten it out so that it is even.

6. Put the dish into the freezer and leave it to set for one hour and a half.

7. Once firm, remove the baking dish from the fridge, slice into 8 chunks and serve.

CAKE BATTER HIGH PROTEIN SMOOTHIE

*Cooking Time: 10 Minutes - Serves: 2 Servings
Calories: 241/Protein: 16 grams/Fiber: 2.5 grams/Fat: 7.6
grams/Carbs: 27.2 grams*

This cake batter smoothie provides all the creamy goodness of a milkshake without the unhealthy ingredients. The two main ingredients in this recipe are bananas and almond milk. Bananas are an excellent source of B6 which plays an important role in mood regulation. Almond milk contains vitamin E which plays a role in wound healing.

Ingredients

- 1 large frozen banana
- 1 cup of almond milk
- ¼ cup of quick oats
- 4 tablespoons of protein powder (vegan)
- 1 tablespoon of cashew butter
- 1 teaspoon of cinnamon
- 1 teaspoon of pure vanilla extract
- ¼ teaspoon of nutmeg

Directions

1. In a small bowl, combine the almond milk and oats.

2. Leave the bowl in the fridge until the oats become soft, this should take around an hour.
3. Add the rest of the ingredients and the oats and milk mixture into a food processor and blend until smooth.
4. Pour into glasses, sprinkle cinnamon over the top and serve.

ZUCCHINI, QUINOA AND CHOCOLATE MUFFINS

*Cooking Time: 40 Minutes - Serves: 9 Servings
Calories: 354/Protein: 14.2 grams/Fiber: 3.7 grams/Fat:
19.4 grams/Carbs: 30.4 grams/Sugar: 19.7 grams*

The unusual ingredient of quinoa in this recipe gives these muffins an extra boost. The two main ingredients in this recipe are quinoa and zucchini. Quinoa is high in calcium which is required for the maintenance of strong bones. Zucchini is a rich source of folate which important when the body is going through periods of rapid growth.

Ingredients

- ½ a cup of dry quinoa
- 2 tablespoons of coconut oil
- 1 ½ cups of almond flour
- ½ a cup of chopped walnuts
- 2 large bananas
- ½ a cup of applesauce
- ¼ cup of maple syrup
- ½ a cup of shredded zucchini
- 1 cup of chocolate or vanilla protein powder (vegan)

- ½ a cup of dark chocolate chips (vegan)
- 5 tablespoons of almond milk
- 2 teaspoons of baking powder
- ½ a teaspoon of cinnamon
- ½ a teaspoon of vanilla extract
- ½ a teaspoon of nutmeg
- A pinch of salt
- ½ a cup of water (optional)

Directions

1. Prepare the quinoa according to the directions on the package and set it to one side.
2. Prepare the oven by preheating it to 400 degrees F.
3. Arrange 8 muffin cups in a baking pan and spray with coconut oil.
4. Combine the baking powder, salt, cinnamon, walnuts, nutmeg and cooked quinoa in a large bowl.
5. In another bowl, combine the applesauce and the bananas and use a fork to mash them together.
6. Add the almond milk, protein powder, maple syrup and the vanilla and stir to combine.
7. Combine the contents of both bowls and stir to combine until a smooth batter has been formed.

8. Add the chocolate chips and the shredded zucchini.
9. Scoop the batter into the muffin cups and fill them halfway.
10. Bake the muffins for 20 minutes until they are fluffy all the way through.
11. Once cooked, remove the muffins from the oven and leave them to cool down before serving.

BROWNIE CHOCOLATE MOCHA BARS

*Cooking Time: 3 Minutes - Serves: 3 Servings
Calories: 213/Protein: 27.3 grams/Fiber: 3.7 grams/Fat: 3.8
grams/Carbs: 17.34 grams/Sugar: 6.1 grams*

You will be overwhelmed by the chocolaty goodness of this bar! The two main ingredients in this recipe are oats and cocoa powder. Oats help to control blood sugar. Cocoa powder is a rich source of polyphenols which helps to reduce blood pressure.

Ingredients
- 2 ½ cups of vanilla or chocolate protein powder
- ½ a cup of cocoa powder
- ½ a cup of quick oats
- 1 teaspoon of pure vanilla extract
- ¼ teaspoon of nutmeg
- 2 tablespoons of agave nectar
- 1 cup of brewed, cold coffee

Directions
1. Lay parchment paper in a baking dish and set it to one side.
2. In a large bowl, combine all the dry ingredients

3. Add the coffee, vanilla extract and agave nectar to the dry ingredients and stir until there are no longer any lumps.
4. Transfer the batter into the dish and make sure you press it into the corners.
5. Put the baking dish into the freezer and freeze for one hour.
6. Once firm, slice and serve.

CHAPTER 11:
IT'S DINNER TIME! WHOLE FOOD MEALS TO AID RECOVERY

SPICY CURRY LENTIL BURGERS

Cooking Time: 1 Hour 20 Minutes - Servings: 12 Servings Calories: 114/Protein: 6 grams/Fat: 1 gram/Carbs: 22 grams

If you want to add a bit of spice to your lentil burger, some curry will do the trick! The two main ingredients in this recipe are lentils and onions. Lentils are an excellent source of protein making them the perfect workout companion. Onions are high in antioxidants which helps the body fight against disease.

Ingredients

- 1 cup of lentils
- 3 cups of water
- 3 grated carrots
- 1 small diced onion
- ¾ cups of whole grain flour
- 2 teaspoons of curry powder
- ½ a teaspoon of sea salt
- A pinch of black pepper
- 12 whole wheat burger buns
- 12 pieces of Romaine lettuce
- 12 slices of tomatoes
- Vega mayonnaise

Directions

1. Boil the lentils in a medium sized saucepan for approximately 30 minutes until they become soft.
2. Place the onion and the carrots in a large bowl, add the salt, pepper, curry powder and flour and toss to combine.
3. Drain the excess water from the lentil and add them to the bowl with the vegetables.
4. Use a potato masher to combine the ingredients, if you need to add more flour, do so.
5. Use your hands to form 12 patties.
6. You can either bake or pan fry the burgers.
7. To bake the burgers, preheat the oven to 350 degrees F.
8. Lay parchment paper on a baking tray and arrange the patties on it.
9. Bake the patties for 499 minutes.
10. Once cooked, remove the patties from the oven.
11. Toast the burger buns and arrange them on plates.
12. Layer with lettuce and tomatoes.
13. Arrange the burgers over the top.
14. Add some mayonnaise, top with the remaining burger bun and serve.

LOADED PIZZA WITH BLACK BEANS

Cooking Time: 30 Minutes - Servings: 2 Servings
Calories: 379/Protein: 13 grams/Fat: 13 grams/Carbs: 59
grams

This awesome healthy pizza will have you coming back for more! The two main ingredients in this recipe are onions and avocado. Onions are a good source of vitamin C which helps to regulate the immune system. Avocado contains riboflavin which assists the body in turning food into energy.

Ingredients
- 2 prebaked pizza crusts
- ½ a cup of spicy black bean dip
- 1 thinly sliced tomato
- A pinch of black pepper
- 1 grated carrot
- A pinch of sea salt
- 1 thinly sliced red onion
- 1 sliced avocado

Directions
1. Preheat the oven to 400 degrees F.
2. Arrange the pizza crusts on a large baking tray.

3. Spread each pizza crust with half of the black bean dip.
4. Arrange the tomato slices over the top and sprinkle with salt.
5. In a small bowl sprinkle the grated carrot with sea salt and use your hands to massage the salt into the carrots.
6. Arrange the carrots over the tomatoes.
7. Spread the onions over the top.
8. Bake the pizza for 20 minutes.
9. Top the pizza with avocado, sprinkle with pepper, slice and serve.

THAI PAD BOWL

Cooking Time: 20 Minutes - Servings: 2 Servings
Calories: 660/Protein: 15 grams/Fat: 19 grams/Carbs: 110
grams

You can whip up this awesome Thai pad recipe in under half an hour! The two main ingredients include brown rice noodles and cabbage. Brown rice noodles contain manganese which plays a role in blood sugar regulation. Cabbage is an excellent source of vitamin C which helps reduce blood pressure.

Ingredients

- 7 ounces of brown rice noodles
- 1 teaspoon of olive oil
- 2 carrots, julienned and peeled
- 1 cup of red cabbage thinly sliced
- 2 finely chopped scallions
- 2 tablespoons of finely chopped fresh mint
- 1 cup of bean sprouts
- ¼ cup of peanut sauce
- ¼ cup of finely chopped cilantro
- 2 tablespoons of chopped roasted peanuts
- Fresh lime wedges

Directions

1. Cook the rice noodles according to the instructions. Once cooked, drain, rinse and set them to one side to cool down.
2. Heat the oil in a large frying pan and sauté the bell pepper, cabbage and carrots for 7 to 8 minutes.
3. Add the bean sprouts, mint and scallions and cook for a further two minutes and take the saucepan off the stove.
4. Combine the vegetables and the noodles and add the peanut sauce.
5. Divide into bowls and sprinkle with peanuts and cilantro.
6. Squeeze the lime wedge over the top and serve.

SUSHI BOWL

*Cooking Time: 20 Minutes - Servings: 1 Servings
Calories: 467/Protein: 22 grams/Fat: 20 grams/Carbs: 56
grams*

This quick and easy sushi bowl makes the perfect mid-week meal. The two main ingredients in this recipe are edamame beans and spinach. Edamame beans are a good source of vitamin K which plays a role in regulating blood calcium levels. Spinach is high in iron which helps support a healthy immune system.

Ingredients

- ½ a cup of fresh edamame beans
- ¼ cup of water
- ¾ cup of cooked brown rice
- ½ a cup of chopped spinach
- ¼ cup of sliced avocado
- ¼ cup of sliced bell pepper
- ¼ cup of chopped fresh cilantro
- 1 chopped scallion
- ¼ nori sheet
- 2 tablespoons of soy sauce
- 1 tablespoon of sesame seeds

Directions

1. Put the edamame beans into a saucepan and steam them with a ¼ cup of water for 15 minutes.
2. Combine the scallions, bell pepper, avocado, spinach, rice and edamame in a bowl and stir to combine.
3. Use a scissors to cut the nori into small pieces and sprinkle it over the top of the vegetables and rice.
4. Drizzle soy sauce over the top and serve.

SWEET POTATO PATTIES

*Cooking Time: 15 Minutes - Servings: 6 Servings
Calories: 146/Protein: 6 grams/Fat: 2 grams/Carbs: 29
grams*

This delightful sweet potato Pattie makes the perfect snack after a long work out. The two main ingredients in this recipe include brown rice and sweet potatoes. Brown rice is considered a low glycemic index food which makes it beneficial for diabetics. Sweet potatoes are packed with fiber which is required for a healthy gut.

Ingredients

- 1 cup of cooked brown rice, short grain, fully cooled
- 1 cup of grated sweet potato
- ½ a cup of chopped onions
- A pinch of sea salt
- ¼ cup of finely chopped fresh parsley
- 1 tablespoon of fresh, chopped dill
- 2 tablespoons of nutritional yeast (optional)
- ½ a cup of whole grain breadcrumbs
- 1 tablespoon of olive oil
- Coconut flour

Directions

1. In a large bowl, combine the onion, sweet potato, rice and salt and stir to combine.
2. Leave the mixture to sit for a couple of minutes to allow the salt to draw out the moisture from the onion and potato.
3. Add the nutritional yeast (if using), dill, parsley and enough flour to make the batter sticky. If you need to add a couple of spoonsful of water.
4. Use your hands to form the mixture into balls, and then flatten them slightly to make patties.
5. Heat the oil in a frying pan and cook the patties for 5 minutes on each side.
6. Remove the patties from the frying pan and serve.

SUMMER VIETNAMESE ROLLS

Cooking Time: 50 Minutes - Servings: 10 Servings
Calories: 77/Protein: 3 grams/Fat: 5 grams/Carbs: 8 grams

Mouthwatering rolls packed with healthy vegetables. The two main ingredients in this recipe are romaine lettuce and carrots. Lettuce is containing potassium which is plays a role in maintaining a healthy nervous system. Carrots are a good source of beta carotene which helps to support the immune system.

Ingredients

- 10 wraps, made from rice roll
- ¼ cup of fresh basil leaves
- 10 Romaine lettuce leaves
- 2 grated carrots
- ½ a julienned cucumber
- 1 mango, peeled and cut into thin, long pieces
- 3 scallions cut into quarters and sliced lengthwise
- 1 cup of bean sprouts
- ½ a cup of peanut sauce

Directions

1. Pour room temperature water into a deep plate.

2. Put one rice roll wrap into the water for a couple of minutes to soften it.
3. Remove it from the water and leave it to drip for a couple of seconds and then place it on a plate.
4. Arrange two fresh basil leaves down the middle of the wrap.
5. Top with a lettuce leaf.
6. Top with bean sprouts, scallions, mango, cucumber and carrots.
7. Fold the bottom and the top of the wrap, fold one side over the filling and push the end under the filling.
8. Use your hand to squeeze the roll slightly and then roll it to the other end.
9. Leave the wraps to sit for a while so that they can stick together.
10. Slice the wraps in half, and serve with peanut sauce for dipping.

SESAME STIR FRY

Cooking Time: 30 Minutes - Servings: 4 Servings
Calories: 334/Protein: 17 grams/Fat: 13 grams/Carbs: 42
grams

A delicious medley of stir-fried vegetables topped with sesame seeds. The two main ingredients in this recipe are quinoa and broccoli. Quinoa is a rich source of magnesium which helps to lower blood pressure. Broccoli is a rich source of potassium helps reduce the risk of diseases such as kidney stones, osteoporosis and stroke.

Ingredients

- 1 cup of quinoa
- 2 cups of water
- A pinch of sea salt
- 1 head of broccoli
- 2 teaspoons of olive oil
- 1 cup of snow peas
- 1 cup of frozen peas
- 2 cups of chopped Swiss chard
- 2 chopped scallions
- 2 tablespoons of water
- 1 teaspoon of toasted sesame oil
- 1 tablespoon of soy sauce
- 2 tablespoons of sesame seeds

Directions

1. In a medium saucepan, add the quinoa, water and sea salt and boil for one minute. Reduce the temperature, put a lid on the saucepan and leave it to simmer for 20 minutes. While the quinoa is cooking, don't stir it.
2. Chop the broccoli up into florets and chop the stem into bite sized pieces.
3. Heat the sesame oil in a frying pan and sauté the broccoli with a pinch of sea salt.
4. Push the broccoli around the pan with a spoon so that it doesn't burn.
5. Add he snow peas and keep stirring, add the scallions and Swiss chard and toss to combine.
6. Add two tablespoons of water to steam the vegetables.
7. Drizzle some sesame oil and soy sauce over the top, toss to combine and remove from the heat.
8. Divide the quinoa into plates, top with the stir fry, sprinkle with sesame seeds and some more soy sauce and serve.

LIME-MINT CREAMY SPAGHETTI SQUASH

*Cooking Time: 40 Minutes - Servings: 3 Servings
Calories: 199/Protein: 7 grams/Fat: 10 grams/Carbs: 27
grams*

If you want to reduce your carbohydrate intake but still feel as if you are eating carbs – this is the recipe for you. The two main ingredients are tahini and lime. Tahini contains more protein than nuts making it the perfect weightlifting companion. Lime is a good source of fiber which assists in the weight loss process because it fills you up faster and keeps you full for longer.

Ingredients for The Dressing

- 3 tablespoons of tahini
- The juice and zest of 1 small lime
- 2 tablespoons of chopped fresh mint
- 1 pressed small clove of garlic
- 1 tablespoon of nutritional yeast
- A pinch of sea salt

Ingredients for The Spaghetti Squash

- 1 spaghetti squash
- A pinch of sea salt
- 1 cup of chopped cherry tomatoes
- 1 cup of bell pepper, chopped
- Ground black pepper

Directions to Make the Dressing

1.   Combine all the ingredients together in a food processor and blend until smooth. Set the dressing to one side.

Directions to Make the Spaghetti Squash

1.   Boil a large pot of water.
2.   Slice the squash in half and used a spoon to scrape the seeds out.
3.   Add salt to the boiling water and boil the squash halves for 30 minutes.
4.   Take the squash out of the pot and leave it to cool down before handling it.
5.   Scoop the squash out and then break apart the strands.
6.   When the squash is boiling it absorbs water and so put the squash noodles into a strainer and leave them to drain for 10 minutes.
7.   Place the spaghetti squash into a bowl and add the dressing.
8.   Top with the bell pepper and cherry tomatoes, sprinkle with black pepper and nutritional yeast (if you are using it) and serve.

PESTO AND SUN-DRIED TOMATO QUINOA

Cooking Time: 15 Minutes - Servings: 1 Serving
Calories: 535/Protein: 20 grams/Fat: 23 grams/Carbs: 69 grams

This recipe is providing a superfood twist to this classic Italian cuisine. The two main ingredients in this recipe are onions and zucchini. Onions contain powerful antioxidants that fight inflammation and reduce cholesterol levels. Zucchini is packed with vitamin C protects the body against cardiovascular disease.

Ingredients

- 1 teaspoon of olive oil
- 1 cup of onion, chopped
- 1 clove of garlic, minced
- 1 cup of zucchini, chopped
- A pinch of sea salt
- 1 chopped tomato
- 2 tablespoons of chopped sun-dried tomatoes
- 3 tablespoons of basil pesto
- 1 cup of chopped spinach
- 2 cups of cooked quinoa
- 1 tablespoon of cheesy sprinkle (optional)

Directions

1. In a large frying pan over a medium temperature, heat the oil.

2. Sauté the onions for 5 minutes.

3. Add the garlic, zucchini and salt and cook for a further 5 minutes.

4. Remove the frying pan from the stove and add the sun-dried and fresh tomatoes and the pesto and toss to combine.

5. Arrange the spinach and quinoa on a plate and top with the zucchini mixture. Top with the cheesy sprinkle (if using).

WHITE BEAN AND OLIVE PASTA

Cooking Time: 10 Minutes - Servings: 1 Serving
Calories: 387/Protein: 18 grams/Fat: 17 grams/Carbs: 42
grams

This delicious pasta is ideal when you are pushed for time. The two main ingredients are whole-grain pasta and red bell pepper. Whole grains are high in fiber which reduces the risk of heart disease. Red bell peppers are an excellent source of vitamin C which helps fight against high blood pressure.

Ingredients

- ½ a cup of whole-grain pasta
- A pinch of sea salt
- 1 teaspoon of olive oil
- ¼ red bell pepper, thinly sliced
- ¼ cup of zucchini, thinly sliced
- ½ cup of cooked cannellini beans
- ½ a cup of spinach
- 1 tablespoon of balsamic vinegar
- 3 black olives, chopped and pitted
- 1 tablespoon of nutritional yeast

Directions

1. Cook the pasta according to the instructions on the packet. Once cooked, drain and rinse and set to one side.

2. Heat the oil in a large saucepan and sauté the zucchini and the bell pepper.
3. Add the beans and cook for 2 minutes.
4. Add the spinach and leave it to wilt.
5. Drizzle the vinegar over the top.
6. Arrange the pasta onto plates, top with the bean mixture, sprinkle the nutritional yeast and the olives over the top and serve.

BUCKWHEAT AND SPAGHETTI MEATBALLS

*Cooking Time: 1 Hour 5 Minutes - Servings: 2 Servings
Calories: 651/Protein: 26 grams/Fat: 15 grams/Carbs: 115
grams*

You will never know you are not eating real meatballs! The two main ingredients in this recipe are buckwheat and flaxseeds. Buckwheat is a good source of protein, the body needs protein to help build bone cartilage. Flaxseeds are high in omega-3 fatty acids which promotes brain health.

Ingredients For the Meatballs
- ½ a cup of toasted buckwheat
- 2 ¼ cups of water
- A pinch of sea salt
- 2 tablespoons of ground flaxseeds
- 2 tablespoons of tomato paste
- 1 tablespoon of stone ground mustard
- 2 tablespoons of soy sauce
- 1 tablespoon of mixed dried herbs
- 1 teaspoon of onion powder
- 1 teaspoon of garlic powder
- ½ a teaspoon of ground cumin
- ½ a teaspoon of smoked paprika

Ingredients For The Spaghetti

- 7 ounces of whole-grain spaghetti
- 2 cups of marinara sauce
- 3 tablespoons of cheesy sprinkle

Directions

1. Prepare the oven by preheating it to 350 degrees F.
2. Grease a baking sheet with olive oil.
3. Add the buckwheat and two cups of water into a small pot, add a pinch of salt and boil it.
4. Reduce the heat, put a lid on the saucepan and leave it to simmer for 5 minutes.
5. Combine the ground flaxseed with ¼ cup of water, stir and set it to one side.
6. In a large bowl, combine the paprika, cumin, garlic powder, onion powder, herbs, soy sauce, mustard and tomato paste and stir to combine.
7. Add the soaked flaxseed and buckwheat and stir to combine.
8. Form the mixture into 2- to 24 small meatballs.
9. Arrange the meatballs onto the baking sheet, and bake for 30 minutes.
10. Cook the spaghetti according to the instructions on the packet; once cooked, drain and rinse it.

11. Remove the meatballs from the oven once they are cooked.
12. Arrange the spaghetti onto plates, top with marinara, meatballs and the cheesy sprinkles and serve.

BLACK EYED PEA BURRITOS

Cooking Time: 50 Minutes - Servings: 6 Servings Calories: 334/Protein: 12 grams/Fat: 6 grams/Carbs: 58 grams

Black eyed pea burritos make a hearty quick meal during the week. The two main ingredients in this recipe are zucchini and black-eyed peas. Zucchini is a rich source of vitamin A which is required for a healthy immune system. Black eyed peas contain copper, the body needs copper to form red blood cells.

Ingredients

- 1 tablespoon of olive oil
- 1 diced red onion
- 2 cloves of minced garlic
- 1 chopped zucchini
- 1 diced and seeded bell pepper
- 1 diced tomato
- 2 tablespoons of chili powder
- A pinch of sea salt
- 1 can of black-eyed peas drained and rinsed
- 6 whole-wheat tortillas

Directions

1. Prepare the oven by preheating it to 350 degrees F.
2. Heat the olive oil in a large frying pan over medium temperature.
3. Sauté the onions for approximately 5 minutes.
4. Add the garlic and continue to sauté for a couple of minutes.
5. Add the zucchini and sauté for five minutes.
6. Add the bell pepper and the tomato and cook for another two minutes.
7. Add the black-eyed peas, salt and chili powder and stir to combine.
8. Lay a tortilla onto a plate and spoon out some of the black-eyed pea mixture into the center. Fold the ends in and roll into a burrito. Repeat for all six burritos.
9. Arrange the burritos seam side down into a baking dish and pour the vegetable juice from the pan over the top.
10. Bake the burritos for 30 minutes. Once cooked, remove from the oven and serve.

CHICKPEA CURRY

*Cooking Time: 15 Minutes - Servings: 2 Servings
Calories: 274/Protein: 10 grams/Fat: 5 grams/Carbs: 49
grams/Fiber: 9 grams*

If you are a curry fan, this meal is for you – bursting with all the spice and flavor you could ever need! The two main ingredients in this recipe are chickpeas and tomato paste. Chickpeas make an excellent meat replacement because of their high protein content. Tomato's contains naringenin which is helps to reduce inflammation in the body.

Ingredients
- Ground black pepper
- The juice of ½ a lemon
- 1 cans of drained and rinsed chickpeas
- 1 tablespoon of maple syrup
- 1/3 cup of tomato paste
- 1 cup of water
- 1 teaspoon of turmeric
- 2 teaspoons of garam masala
- 2 teaspoons of ground cumin
- 2 teaspoons of ground coriander
- 1 tablespoon of chili powder
- 1 tablespoon of fresh minced ginger

- Salt
- 1 chopped onion
- 1 tablespoon of olive oil
- 2 cups of brown rice

Directions

1. Cook the brown rice according to the instructions on the packet and set to one side.
2. In a medium sized frying pan, heat the oil over medium heat.
3. Add the onions and a pinch of salt, stir until the onions become soft.
4. Add the ginger and garlic and cook for another 1 minute.
5. Add the garam masala, cumin, coriander and chili powder, stir to combine and cook for another 1 minute.
6. Add the chickpeas, maple syrup, tomato paste, water and some salt, stir to combine, place a lid over the pan, reduce the temperature to low and leave the ingredients to simmer for 10 minutes.
7. Add the lemon juice and black pepper and stir to combine.
8. Spoon the brown rice out onto dishes, top with the curry and serve.

SWEET POTATO SHEPHARD'S PIE

Cooking Time: 1 Hour 10 Minutes - Servings: 6 Servings Calories: 189/Protein: 9 grams/Fat: 3 grams/Carbs: 32 grams/Fiber: 6 grams

A classic comfort food with a healthy spin! The two main ingredients in this recipe are sweet potatoes and lentils. Sweet potatoes are an excellent source of pantothenic acid which is required to help the body convert food into energy. Lentils are rich in iron. The body needs iron to transport oxygen to the blood.

Ingredients

- Coarsely chopped parsley
- 1 teaspoon of smoked paprika
- 2 tablespoons of tamari
- 3 tablespoons of tomato paste
- 1 teaspoon of garlic powder
- ¼ cup of unsweetened almond milk
- 2 medium sized sweet potatoes
- 2 ½ cups of vegetable broth
- 1 cup of brown lentils
- 3 cloves of minced garlic
- Salt
- 2 stalks of finely chopped celery
- 1 finely chopped carrot

- 1 finely chopped onion
- 1 tablespoon of coconut oil

Directions

1. Heat the oil in a medium sized saucepan and add the celery, carrot, onion and a pinch of salt. Stir to combine and cook for about 1 minute.
2. Add the garlic and cook for a further 1 minute.
3. Add the vegetable broth and the lentils and bring to a boil. Let the ingredients simmer for 30 minutes.
4. Steam the potatoes in for 10 minutes in a steamer basket. Once they are soft, transfer the potatoes into a medium sized bowl.
5. Add the garlic powder and the milk and a pinch of salt. Use a potato masher to mash the potatoes and combine the mixture together.
6. Once the tomatoes are cooked, add the smoked paprika, Tamari and tomato paste and stir to combine.
7. Pour the lentils into a baking dish, top with a layer of the sweet mashed potatoes and bake for 15 minutes until the top becomes crisp.
8. Remove the dish from the oven, garnish with fresh parsley and serve.

STOVETOP MAPLE BEANS

*Cooking Time: 20 Minutes - Servings: 6 Servings
Calories: 364/Protein: 19 grams/Fat: 3 grams/Carbs: 67
grams/Fiber: 19 grams*

Add some Smokey sweetness to your dinner plate with these finger-licking stovetop maple beans. The two main ingredients in this recipe are white navy beans and tomatoes. White navy beans are a good source of manganese which is required for blood sugar regulation. Tomatoes contain vitamin K which is required for the maintenance of healthy bones.

Ingredients

- Ground black pepper
- 1 teaspoon of smoked paprika
- 1 teaspoon of Dijon mustard
- 2 teaspoons of apple cider vinegar
- 1 tablespoon of tamari
- 2 tablespoons of fancy molasses
- 3 tablespoons of maple syrup
- 1 can of diced tomatoes
- 7 cups of white navy beans
- 3 cloves of minced garlic
- Salt
- 1 stalk of finely chopped celery

- 1 finely chopped carrot
- 1 finely chopped onion
- 1 tablespoon of olive oil
- Rosemary parsley protein

Directions

1. In a large stockpot, heat the oil over a medium temperature.
2. Add the celery, carrots and onions and sauté until the onions become translucent.
3. Add the garlic and cook for a further one minute.
4. Add the paprika, mustard, apple cider vinegar, aminos, molasses, syrup, tomatoes and beans and stir to combine.
5. Serve the beans with rosemary parsley protein bread.

CABBAGE ROLL STEW

*Cooking Time: 50 Minutes - Servings: 6 Servings
Calories: 211/Protein: 10 grams/Fat: 3 grams/Carbs: 36
grams/Fiber: 7 grams*

This hearty protein rich stew is the perfect choice for anyone wanting to shed a few pounds. The two main ingredients in this recipe are brown rice and tomatoes. Brown rice is a rich source of fiber which facilitates the digestion process. Tomatoes contain folate which is required for making red and white blood cells.

Ingredients

- 2 cups of brown rice
- Chopped parsley for garnish
- 2 tablespoons of apple cider vinegar
- 1 coarsely chopped cabbage
- 1 can of diced tomatoes
- 3 cups of vegetable broth
- 2 teaspoons of dried thyme
- 1 cup of dried brown lentils
- 2 cups of chopped brown mushrooms
- 2 cloves of minced garlic
- Salt
- 1 chopped onion
- 1 tablespoon of olive oil

Directions

1. Cook the brown rice according to the directions on the packet and set to one side.
2. Heat the oil in a large stockpot over medium heat.
3. Add the onions and a pinch of salt and cook until the onions become translucent.
4. Add the mushrooms and garlic and cook for a further 5 minutes.
5. Add the broth, thyme and lentils and let the ingredients boil. Turn the heat down to low, put a lid on the stockpot and leave it to simmer for 25 minutes.
6. Add the vinegar, cabbage, tomatoes and some salt and cook for a further five minutes.
7. Divide the rice onto plates, spoon the cabbage stew over the top, garnish with parsley and serve.

CHAPTER 12:
LET'S GET SAUCY - FLAVOR BOOSTERS AND SAUCES FOR EXCITING MEALS

BECHAMEL SAUCE

Cooking Time: 10 Minutes - Serves: 2 Cups
Calories: 105 /Protein: 3.8 grams/Fiber: 0.1 grams/Fat: 7 grams/Carbs: 7 grams

Bechamel sauce is an absolute requirement for every home cook!

Ingredients

- 3 tablespoons of vegan butter
- 2 tablespoons of flour
- 2 cups of war milk (non-dairy)
- Salt and pepper
- A pinch of nutmeg (if you like)

Directions

1. In a saucepan over medium temperature melt the butter.
2. Add the flour and whisk until it starts to bubble and thicken, make sure it doesn't start browning, this should take about 2 minutes.
3. Add the warm milk into the pan and keep whisking until the sauce starts to thicken even more, this should take about 3 minutes.
4. Add the nutmeg (if you are using it), salt and pepper and stir to combine.

5. If you are not going to use the sauce straight away, place wax paper over it until you are ready to use the sauce.

CARAMEL SAUCE

Cooking Time: 5 Minutes - Serves: 1
Calories: 75 /Fat: 2.4 grams/Carbs: 14 grams

This seriously delicious, dreamy, and creamy caramel sauce is going to drive you insane. The two main ingredients in this recipe are agave syrup and almond butter. Agave syrup is low in fat and low in calories making it the perfect weight loss companion. Almond butter is an excellent source of magnesium which helps to boost exercise performance.

Ingredients

- 1 teaspoon of water
- 1 tablespoon of agave syrup
- 1 tablespoon of almond butter

Directions

1. Put all the ingredients into a small bowl and whisk to combine.
2. Set it to one side for a few minutes to thicken up.

CHEESE CASHEW MOZZARELLA SAUCE

*Cooking Time: 1 Hour 25 Minutes - Serves: 2 Cups
Calories: 98 /Protein: 2.3 grams/Fiber: 0.9 grams/Fat:
grams/Carbs: 7.6 grams*

This melty, stringy vegan mozzarella sauce will fool the most diligent cheese connoisseur. The two main ingredients in this recipe are cashews and lemon juice. Cashews contain monounsaturated fats which are required for the maintenance of heart health. Lemon juice is high in vitamin C helps to protect the cells and keep them healthy.

Ingredients

- 1 ½ cups of raw cashews
- 1 cup of water
- 2 tablespoons of corn starch
- 2 tablespoons of lemon juice

Directions

1. Put the cashews in a bowl of water and soak them overnight.
2. Transfer all the ingredients into a food processor and blend until they become smooth.
3. The sauce will last for 3 days in the fridge, but it will last for one month if frozen.

SPICY CHEESE SAUCE

Cooking Time: 10 Minutes - Serves: 2 Cups
Calories: 418/Protein: 3 grams/Fat: 8 grams/Carbs:4 grams

This simple sauce tastes better when it's made without cheese, but tastes just like cheese! The two main ingredients in this recipe are cashews and nutritional yeast. Cashews are high in vitamin E which is required for the maintenance of healthy eyes and skin. Nutritional yeast is an excellent source of vitamin B12 which is required for red blood cell formation.

Ingredients
- 1 cup of raw cashews
- 1 garlic clove
- ½ a cup of nutritional yeast
- 1/3 cup of water
- 2 tablespoons of extra virgin olive oil
- ½ a teaspoon of paprika
- ¼ teaspoon of Chipotle pepper powder
- ½ a teaspoon of sea salt
- 1 teaspoon of cumin

Directions
1. Put the cashew nuts into a bowl and soak them overnight.
2. Transfer all the ingredients into a food processor and blend until creamy and smooth.

CHILI GREEN NACHO SAUCE

Cooking Time: 10 Minutes - Serves: 2 Cups
Calories: 78 /Protein: 1.5 grams/Fiber: 0.8 grams/Fat: 5
grams/Carbs: 7 grams

This chili green sauce is incredibly versatile, you can drizzle it over warm cauliflower, broccoli, roasted vegetables or use it as a dip. The two main ingredients in this recipe are cashews and green chilis. Cashews are a rich source of potassium which helps to boost metabolism and enhance muscle strength. Green chilis are rich in vitamin C which is required for healthy skin rejuvenation.

Ingredients

- 1 cup of raw cashews
- ¼ cup of diced red roasted peppers
- ½ cup of diced green chilis
- 2 tablespoons of nutritional yeast flakes
- 2 teaspoons of lemon juice
- 1 cup of water
- ½ a teaspoon of cayenne pepper
- ½ a teaspoon of sea salt

Directions

1. Put the cashews into a bowl of water and leave them to soak overnight.
2. Transfer all the ingredients into a food processor and blend until smooth.

WORCESTERSHIRE SAUCE

Cooking Time: 7 Minutes - Serves: 2 Cups
Calories: 6/Protein: 0.00 grams/Carbs: 0.90 grams

This delicious plant-based home cooked version tastes better than any other Worcestershire sauce you will ever taste! The two main ingredients in this recipe are lemon and cider vinegar. Lemon is high in vitamin C which supports the immune system. Cider vinegar contains probiotics which maintain gut health.

Ingredients
- 1 cup of cider vinegar
- 1/3 cup of dark molasses
- ¼ cup of tamari
- ¼ cup of water
- 3 tablespoons of lemon juice
- 1/8 teaspoon of ground cardamom
- 1/8 teaspoon of ground cloves
- ¼ teaspoon of ground cinnamon
- ¼ teaspoon of cayenne pepper
- ¼ teaspoon of garlic powder
- ½ a teaspoon of black pepper
- ¾ teaspoon of ground ginger
- 1 teaspoon of onion powder

- ½ a tablespoon of dry mustard powder
- 1 ½ tablespoons of salt
- A sterilized pint jar

Directions

1. Transfer all the ingredients into a food processor and blend until combined.
2. Transfer the mixture into a medium sized saucepan and boil.
3. Take the saucepan from the heat and pour the mixture into a sterilized pint jar.
4. You can store the sauce in the fridge for up to seven days.

TZATZIKI

Cooking Time: 10 Minutes - Serves: 2 Cups
Calories: 50 /Protein: 2 grams/Fiber: 1 gram/Fat: 3.5
grams/Carbs: 3 grams

You will recognize this sauce as that delicious yogurt and cucumber sauce you always find at Greek restaurants! This chilled and refreshing recipe can be used as a spread or a dip. The two main ingredients in this recipe are cucumber and vegan yogurt. Cucumbers are high in antioxidants which protect the body against oxidative stress. Vegan yogurt is full of probiotics which help to maintain gut health.

Ingredients
- 1 cup of plain vegan yogurt
- ¼ grated cucumber
- 1 tablespoon of fresh dill
- 1 tablespoon of lemon juice
- 1 tablespoon of olive oil
- 1 clove of minced garlic
- 1 teaspoon of salt
- 1 teaspoon of black pepper
- 1 tablespoon of nutritional yeast
- 1 teaspoon of lemon zest

Directions

1. Transfer all the ingredients into a food processor and blend until completely smooth.
2. Pour the mixture out into a bowl, cover and leave it to chill in the fridge for an hour before serving. For better flavor, leave it in the fridge overnight.

VEGAN FISH SAUCE

Cooking Time: 10 Minutes/Serves: 2 Cups
Calories: 3.1 /Protein: 0.3 grams/Fiber: 0.1 grams/Carbs:
0.5 grams

This amalgamation of very intense flavors makes for the perfect sauce over any Asian style dish of your choice. The main ingredients in this recipe are mushrooms and wakame. Mushrooms are high in the powerful antioxidant selenium which prevents damage to the cells and tissues and helps to support the immune system.

Ingredients

- 1/3 cup of dark soy sauce, mushroom flavored
- 1 teaspoon of whole peppercorns
- 2 large cloves of garlic, crushed
- 2 cups of filtered water
- ½ a cup of shredded wakame
- 1 teaspoon of genmai miso

Directions

1. In a large saucepan, combine the peppercorns, garlic and wakame, bring the ingredients to a boil, reduce the heat and leave it to simmer for 20 minutes.

2. Strain the liquid and then pour it back into the saucepan.
3. Add the soy sauce and let the ingredients boil again until the liquid has reduced to half and it tastes extremely salty.
4. Take the saucepan from the heat, add the miso and stir to combine.
5. Leave the sauce to cool down completely.
6. Pour the cooled sauce into a bottle and store in the fridge.

SATAY PEANUT SAUCE

*Cooking Time: 10 Minutes - Serves: 2 Cups
Calories: 45 /Protein: 1 gram/Fiber: 0.4 grams/Fat: 4
grams/Carbs: 1 gram*

Whip up this easy to make peanut sauce in 10 minutes! It makes a delicious dip for vegetable skewers and party nibbles. The two main ingredients in this recipe are peanuts and shallots. Peanuts are a rich source of phosphorous which is required to filter waste from the kidneys.

Ingredients

- The juice of 1 lemon
- 1 ¾ cups of water
- 2 ½ tablespoons of water
- 1 tablespoon of dark soy sauce
- ½ a teaspoon of soft brown sugar
- ½ a teaspoon of chili powder
- Salt
- 4 chopped shallots
- 1 clove of chopped garlic
- 1 ½ cups of raw peanuts with the skin
- 1/3 cup of peanut oil
- 2 ¾ tablespoons of peanut oil

Directions

1. Heat the oil in a wok and cook the peanuts for five minutes. Remove the peanuts from the wok using a slotted spoon to drain the oil and set them to one side. Save 1 tablespoon of oil and pour out the rest.
2. Once the peanuts have cooled down, grind them in a coffee grinder or a food processor if you don't have one.
3. Crush the shallots, garlic and a pinch of salt in a mortar and then fry in the wok with the reserved oil for 1 minute.
4. Add the rest of the ingredients except the peanuts and the lemon juice and bring to a boil.
5. Add the ground peanuts and leave the ingredients to simmer for 10 minutes stirring every so often until the sauce gets thicker.
6. Add a pinch of salt, the lemon juice and take the wok off the stove.
7. If you are not going to use the sauce straight away, leave it to cool down completely, and then store the sauce in an airtight jar in the fridge for up to a week. When you are ready to use it, heat the sauce before serving.

HONEY SPICY MUSTARD

Cooking Time: 10 Minutes - Serves: 2 Cups
Calories: 150 /Protein: 1 gram/Fat: 9 grams/Carbs: 16
grams

A spicy sauce to spread over sandwiches, use as a dip for fries, cauliflower wings or dish that you prefer. The two main ingredients in this recipe include brown rice syrup and mustard. Brown rice syrup is high in fiber which helps to maintain bowl health. Mustard contains calcium which is required for the nerves, muscles and heart to function properly.

Ingredients

- ½ a cup of vegan mayonnaise
- 1 tablespoon of Dijon mustard
- 3 tablespoons of brown rice syrup
- 1 teaspoon of red wine vinegar
- ¼ teaspoon of cayenne pepper
- 1/8 teaspoon of chili powder

Preparation

1. Transfer all the ingredients into a food processor and blend to combine.
2. Pour into a container and store in the fridge for up to one week.

CONCLUSION

Congratulations! You have got to the end of the book! I hope you have enjoyed reading every page, and that you have at least started making some of the recipes. But before you go, I would just like to remind you that if you are diligent about following the recipes in this book, you will achieve your ideal body. Contrary to popular belief, diet plays an essential role in manipulating your physique. You can do a 1000 sit ups per day and gain some definition, but if that muscle tone is surrounded by fat, no one is going to see it.

There are so many delicious and satisfying meals in this cookbook that will not only fuel your training, but will also get you shredded and jacked, and every single recipe is 100 percent dairy free and meatless!

There is a huge misconception that we've got to eat meat to get protein. There are plenty of plant-based foods that contain a higher percentage of protein than meat. Think about it, there are several vegetarian animals; in fact, some of the most powerful beasts in the animal kingdom such as rhinos, elephants and gorillas don't eat meat, so where do they get their protein from? In the plants they eat! So, it is more than possible for plant-based dieters to get more than enough protein to support their workout goals.

The key with any diet is consistency, going plant-based shouldn't be something you do just to meet your fitness goals – it should become a lifestyle!

I wish you every success on your journey to plant based wholeness!

* 9 7 9 8 6 1 5 3 0 4 8 3 5 *